Dear Food,
I love you.
I hate you.
Don't leave me!

Dear Food,
I love you.
I hate you.
Don't leave me!

A Bible study program designed to help you shatter
food strongholds for lasting health and joy

By Julia Fikse, NBC-HWC, FMCHC

Nationally Board-Certified Health and Wellness Coach
Functional Medicine Certified Health Coach
Specialized Certifications in Weight Loss, and Mental Health & Emotional Eating

Bible verses are pulled from BibleHub.com.

Front cover cake photo by Craig Fikse.

ISBN: 979-8-218-01551-0 PAPERBACK

ISBN: 979-8-218-01552-7 EBOOK

For more information go to www.onesteptowellness.com

Dedication

For you, Lord Jesus.
Thank you. I love you.

Acts 4:12
Psalm 23
John 15:5

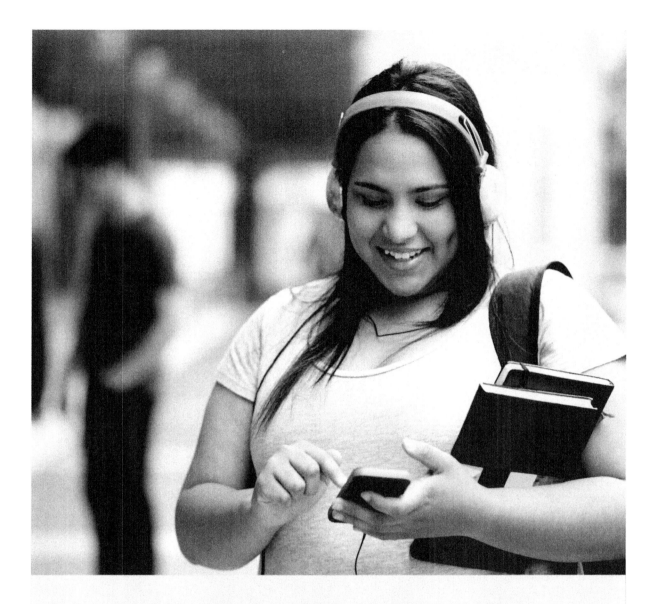

GET THE DEAR FOOD
FREE DIGITAL CONTENT:
PLAYLIST
CHAPTER VIDEOS
...AND MORE

www.onesteptowellness.com

Contents

How to Use This Program

1. This program is designed to be used in a small group Bible Study setting. You can do it on your own; however, you will find it most meaningful and effective surrounded by and sharing with people who are going through the same struggle.

2. It's best to work the program in order, both by chapter and book. Each book provides material for a 10-week Bible Study, and there are three books in the series. This is Book One.

3. The series fits into the Fall, Winter, and Spring Bible study rotation format used in many churches. Fall Session=Book 1, Winter Session=Book 2, and Spring Session= Book 3, with a break for summer. Find and/or request worksheets available for download at: www.onesteptowellness.com

4. Please begin by reading "My Food Story." If you are meeting with a group, please ask the group to read "My Food Story" before the first meeting.

5. This program was written with those who are already Christ-followers in mind. If you are not yet a Christ-follower I recommend:

    a. Working this program with a group who loves Jesus
    b. Reading the following before you start:
        i. One or all of gospels Matthew, Mark, Luke, and John, the first books in the New Testament (I recommend John in the New Living Translation)
        ii. *The Case for Christ*, by Lee Strobel
        iii. *The New Testament Documents, Are They Reliable?* By FF Bruce

    Once you know Jesus, understand how much He loves you, and have the Holy Spirit in your heart, this program will be a completely different experience.

6. For best results, invite Jesus to be a part of your journey. If you're not sure how to ask or what to pray, you can use this prayer to start. In time, your own prayers will come.

    Dear Jesus, I invite you to join me as I study the Bible today and learn more about you, my body, and food. Please come and sit with me, teach me, and give me wisdom. I can't wait to see your goodness unfold. Open the eyes of my heart, and help me see you, hear you, and follow you. Amen.

    "If any of you lacks wisdom, you should ask God, who gives generously to all without finding fault, and it will be given to you." (James 1:5 NIV)

7. Use the Bible as your number one guide for life. While I sincerely hope my words will encourage and help you, I am only human. The Word of God contains the ultimate words to live by.

8. The goal of this program is to invite you into a deeper and more meaningful relationship with the Lord, create space for you to discover the root cause(s) of your struggle with unhealthy eating, and help you design *your own* meaningful strategies for building health and joy—strategies that work for you because *you* created them. Your life experience and your relationship with food are unique, and therefore you are the best person to determine your action steps. In this program, creating those steps, and taking them, is exclusively up to you.

9. Eating is an important part of life and health. This program is about identifying and learning to stop 1) *unhealthy and harmful* eating and 2) *unhealthy and harmful* eating practices. No part of this book should be interpreted to mean any person should unsafely restrict or stop eating.

10. This book is not intended to be psychotherapy or to diagnose, treat, or cure any illness, physical or mental. Yet, as with any journey of self-discovery, unresolved trauma or health concerns may surface. This program is not a substitute for counseling, psychotherapy, psychoanalysis, mental health care, substance abuse treatment, nutrition advice, or a doctor's care. *Please seek professional help if you need it.* And just in case, if at any time you begin to experience self-harming thoughts or activities (for example: anorexia, bulimia, cutting, suicidal ideation), please seek professional help immediately, call 911, or call the National Suicide Prevention Hotline (1-800-273-8255). Life can be very hard and leave us with serious emotional and even physical scars. Getting professional help may be just what you need to thrive.

11. Before you begin, let go of past disappointments and forget past failures. God is doing a new thing, and nothing can stop the wonderful work He is doing in you. Where there is no way, God makes a way. Start this new journey anticipating exciting revelations and victories you never dreamed possible.

"Anyone who belongs to Christ is a new person. The past is forgotten, and everything is new."
2 Corinthians 5:17

"See, I am doing a new thing! Now it springs up; do you not perceive it? I am making a way in the wilderness and streams in the wasteland."
Isaiah 43:19

My prayer for you:

"God of our Lord Jesus the Anointed, Father of Glory: I call out to You on behalf of Your people. Give them minds ready to receive wisdom and revelation so they will truly know You. Open the eyes of their hearts, and let the light of Your truth flood in. Shine Your light on the hope You are calling them to embrace. Reveal to them the glorious riches You are preparing as their inheritance. Let them see the full extent of Your power that is at work in those of us who believe, and may it be done according to Your might and power." Ephesians 1:17–19 (VOICE version)

It's time to discover your path to lasting health, vitality and joy.

This is so exciting! Let's do it.

But first, here is "My Food Story". I share it so you know this program has been created with humility and a personal understanding of what it's like to fight unhealthy food and unhealthy food behaviors for a lifetime. You are not alone.

My Food Story

The Day This Book Almost Didn't Happen
January 7, 2018: 46 years old

The winter sun streamed through our window, and I cracked open my eyes, hoping a good night's rest had soothed my symptoms. No change. Chills, fatigue, nausea, and fever persisted. What was I doing wrong?

Exactly one week earlier, on New Year's Eve, I checked into the ER because of severe gut pain. After an ultrasound and bloodwork, I was sent home, and there was no follow-up, so I went about life, powering through this crazy bug. I returned to the clinic on Friday because my neighbor, a doctor, eyes deep with concern, told me my skin looked gray and to "go back." They took more blood, sent me home, and prescribed antibiotics. What else could I do?

My husband stirred next to me as I shuffled to the bathroom. Something wasn't right. Heading back to bed, a firework exploded in my belly, and I fell to the ground. My husband called 911. Why couldn't I stand up? Hot pain flooded my body.

I still see the dusty black boots and reflective hems on khaki canvas marching across our carpet. I hear men's voices asking me questions I couldn't answer between vomiting and internal organ agony. Was the road to the hospital always this bumpy? The ER staff were sure I had the flu. "No. It's not the flu." I whimpered. Since I was vomiting with a fever, they disregarded my self-diagnosis and put me in the waiting room with other flu victims for six hours. My husband tried to tell them it wasn't the flu. Why wouldn't they listen to us? I was so weak; even though I wanted to speak up, I couldn't. Finally, they took a group of us "with the flu" to a large room near triage. A doctor came in and surveyed all the patients waiting for a bed. She took one look at me, pointed, and demanded, "Give that one a bed. NOW."

My body rejected everything I swallowed, including oral medication, so I was given an IV. A surgeon marched around hurling orders, "Why hasn't she been given the contrast yet?" and "What are you waiting for? Now!" Then he'd leave, powered by the smoke bursting out of his ears. The young, cheerful nurse next to me started shaking and wouldn't meet my eyes. Did he scare her?

The doctor who picked me out of the crowd for a room resurfaced, put her hand on my arm, looked me in the eyes, and told me the following:

1) I was septic.
2) My organs had not shut down yet—but it wouldn't be long.
3) There wasn't much time.
4) She had never "lost anyone" on her watch, and that wasn't going to start today.

She explained that the surgeon needed to see what was going on in my body via CAT scan and ordered contrast that was typically swallowed. Since I wasn't keeping anything down, they would administer it through an NG tube. They would do it now, it was going to be unpleasant, and it would take two nurses.

Nasogastric Intubation: Inserting a plastic tube through the nose, down the esophagus, and into the stomach.

The tube was heftier than I anticipated. I prayed for endurance and let them attempt insertion. Since it's not a common procedure, it took two tries. As they were jabbing the device into my body through my nose, I began to grasp the gravity of my situation.

The CAT scan explained nothing. They had no choice but to cut me open and attempt to locate the problem on the operating table.

There was a very real possibility at this point I would die.
I could lose my colon and live out my days with a colostomy bag.
I could have serious organ damage.

The surgeon was tasked with going into surgery blind in an attempt to save my life. I was wheeled into prep as his gruff voice demanded, "Faster!" and "There is no time!"

Flying through the cold, dark hall on a cold hospital bed, my husband paced alongside, holding my hand. We shared our love and remembered moments of life together. We prayed, and he kissed me. I asked him to tell the kids not to blame God if I died because even though bad things happen in this world, God is good. He nodded and after fighting for me all day long, he could go no farther. I was thrust through swinging doors, over the threshold into an emergency surgery that would alter my life forever.

Welcome!

Hi. My name is Julia, and I love food. Nice to meet you!

Thankfully, that was not the end of my story, and I can't wait to tell you what God did. But first, we came here to talk about our tumultuous relationship with food and how to overcome eating strongholds that separate us from health and joy.

Let's do it.

If you're reading this, you probably also love food, but food has stopped loving you back. You're asking yourself, "How did I get stuck in these frustrating food patterns again?" and "Will I ever break free?"

Together we're going to discover how to finally experience greater victory than you ever thought possible.

This book *is not* about "how you look" or "what you weigh." You are valuable and loved as you are (even though some of you may find that hard to believe at the moment).

This book *is* about discovering why you can't stop unhealthy eating and/or food behavior(s) though you try without end and try again. No matter your food challenge, whether it is overeating, sugar addiction, restricting, binging, purging, or (fill in the blank,) this book is about taking hold of the victories you so desperately seek—and holding on to them for life.

Although many report losing weight while doing the program, this won't be our focus. Instead, we will explore our emotional, mental, and spiritual attachment to food so that we can discover effective solutions, peace, and wellness that lasts. The bathroom scale is no measure of our heart or our emotional and mental well-being. In fact, I would argue that at times the bathroom scale may be more damaging than it is helpful for many people.

For now, we are not going to focus on "losing." In fact, this book is about increase—gaining hope, growing peace, putting on wisdom, and adding experience trusting the Lord with your food and your body. As you go through this material, you will come to comprehend your value as the Lord's precious child and connect the dots between your worth, your purpose, your body, and how you consume food.

Many suffer in silence under the devastating oppression of food. If you do as well, you're not alone. I've been there, and that is why I have written this material. It's my hope that through this study, you will discover a large community of new friends who you can relate to and who can encourage you, a Savior who deeply cares about your food challenges because He loves you, and countless new and exciting successes that make your heart soar.

If you are ready to overthrow the power food has over you, this book is for you. It will be an inspiring, rewarding, and life-changing journey with the Lord as our leader.

How do I know this is possible? I have lived through a life-long fierce battle with food, and Jesus saved me and changed me. It is my prayer that in telling you my food story, you will have hope that He can do the same for you and renew your confidence that victory is possible with Jesus at the helm.

This is my food story.

I Can Do It Myself
1977: 5 Years Old

My mom came into my room to kiss me goodnight and asked if I would like to ask Jesus into my heart.

"Yes," I replied.
"Would you like me to pray with you?"
"No, I'll do it myself," I said.
"Are you sure?"
"I can do it myself,"

"OK." She kissed my head and left.

I asked Jesus into my heart that night, was given the precious gift of the Holy Spirit and became a part of God's family. Although I was only five, it is the single best decision I've ever made, and I did it myself.

We lived on a twisty street in the Oakland hills. There were no sidewalks, only hairpin curves covered in pine needles and eucalyptus branches that crunched under tires weaving around every bend.

It was the morning of the big elementary concert in the gym. The fog hovered low, gifting a blanket of cover and cool that wouldn't burn off till late afternoon. The kindergartners were performing, and my mom dropped me off in a pink, puffy dress with frills. As I walked through the chain link fence into the misty play yard, I noticed that not one other girl was fancy. I panicked and ran out to catch my mom before she drove away, but the lot was empty.

I started home on foot.

Cars raced by me around turns. I kept walking. A rope separated me from a steep cliff on the right that ended in a damp gulch of sharp rocks below. I marched on. Someone pulled over, grabbed me, and dragged me to their car. I kicked, took a bite, was released, and ran.

My mother answered my knock, whisked me into play clothes and drove me right back to school.

Standing on the risers that day, surrounded by girls in puffy dresses with frills, I realized I may have misjudged my situation.

But I walked home, all by myself.

Even at a young age, I remember being too proud to ask for or accept help. The characteristic would blossom, at times for good and at others to my detriment. It was my "I can do it myself" core value that would spiral my relationship with food and lock me in a secret, internal prison of chaotic eating that pride did not allow me to reveal to anyone.

It's just food. I should be able to handle it all by myself, right?

Boys and Body Image
1980: 8 Years Old

He was a blonde-haired rebel in a torn, tie-dyed t-shirt. Lively, loud, and leading the pack, he sprinted by me at week-away camp flanked by friends. Flashing a smile in my direction, he shouted, "Hey, pig legs!"

In a cloud of dust and dirt, he was gone … and with him went my self-esteem.

I did not comfortably wear shorts or skirts again until my late-40s.

The First Time Food Broke My Heart
1987: 15 Years Old

It was the mid-80s, and if you survived the decade of big bangs, front pleats, and gulping down hot hose water from a dirty brass nozzle, you know three things ruled: summer, Saturday morning cartoons, and sugar cereal "fortified with 12 essential vitamins and minerals." (Fortified = healthy, right?)

The time had come to leave my second-generation home video game console behind and hit the road in our wood-paneled green station wagon. Destination: week-away camp. Sitting on the rear-facing bench in the "way back" with no seatbelt, weaving plastic lanyards, and yelling "Are we there yet?" was a dream come true for me, maybe not for my parents. Ahhh, the smell of hot vinyl in July.

I peeled my skin off the seat and waved goodbye as the dust kicked up and swirled behind their rear tires. Inhaling the glorious scent of dirt, pine, and freedom, I galloped off to claim a top bunk.

One Week Later …

Sprinting to my mom at pick up, dragging a half-stuffed sleeping bag on the trail behind me, I watched her expression morph from welcome to shock. She hugged me, tried to collect herself, and asked absently if I remembered my pillow. When we got in the car and closed the door, the real question surfaced … How did I gain so much weight in one week?

Unlimited soft-serve access. That's how.

I rambled on about camp all the way home trying to avoid my mother's eyes. You'd think from *listening* to me that my best friend at camp (and new pen pal) was a girl named Amy—fun, pretty, and mercurial. You'd know from *looking* at me that my best friend at camp that week was swirly soft ice cream—fun, pretty, and also … mercurial.

Next thing I knew, we were home, and Mom was teaching me how to count calories. Obesity runs in our family, and she had good reason to be concerned. To me, the "food limits" felt like punishment. I was ashamed, and my heart ached.

Food did this to me, and I would NEVER let food hurt me again. EVER.

Maybe Not Never

Over the next four years, I would diet to eat and eat because I could diet. My beauty ideals were Princess Diana and the senior girl in choir who was so thin she could sit cross-legged in a miniskirt and wrap her top leg all the way around her bottom leg with a twist and flap her flat shoes against the bottom of her feet with her toes. Wow—I longed to be so thin I could wrap my top leg around my bottom leg like a pretzel, flap my flats … and eat whatever I wanted, whenever I wanted it. Was that *really* too much to ask?

My high school self was fueled by the need to get good grades, have good friends, and eat good food. If the first two didn't work out, the third always came through. If I was dieting, life was dull, unbearable, and filled with headaches. When I was not dieting, I was making up for lost time, numbing out on food and gaining weight fast.

And so the vicious cycle of binging, weight gain, shame, restricting, starving, binging, weight gain, shame, restricting and starving took root. But I could handle it myself. It's just food. Calories in calories out, right?

Lunch was not cafeteria fries for me. I wasn't born with the kind of body that can process fried, junky, cool-kids food and stay thin. (This simple fact alone caused me to harbor resentment and bitterness I buried with chocolate for decades.) My "lunch" was a couple of crackers, a few pieces of cheese, and maybe if I was feeling thin, an apple. My mom was a good cook and cared about providing healthy meals. We ate dinner as a family, with proper portions for all. How then, you might ask, did I gain weight?

Eating to soothe after school. Eating for a boost while studying. Eating to zone out with Thursday TV, followed by "Cheat Day" Friday that led to "Why Not Saturday" and "Oh Well I Already Blew It Sunday." My body expanded as I solidified the habit of eating to regulate the ever-changing emotional landscape of life.

I was skilled at managing school, work and relationships… if I could temper it all, devastating or delightful, with food.

Babysitting kept the cash and snacks flowing. I picked homes where the family said, "Help yourself to whatever food you can find." If you insist. I was a good babysitter, a kind and responsible girl who loved the Lord and took care of their kiddos. I also did the dishes and picked up. Who would notice (or care) if I ate half a carton of ice cream topped with the last of the mini marshmallows? Cloaked in the shadow and stillness of someone else's home with the children snoring, the TV flickering, and permission to eat … I disassociated my binge eating in the dark from my actual life in the light of day. Denial had its hooks in me. If you eat nachos in someone else's house in the dark, calories don't count, right?

After a weekend of babysitting and binging, Mondays meant harsh restricting, and I was moody, frustrated, and fatigued. I hated Monday. It was "my diet starts today" day. I was so disgusted with myself that I didn't allow much in the way of nutrition. After dinner, homework, and chores, I gave in to the goodies after a long day of raging food battles in my mind. I'd wake up Tuesday morning, "Beat It" blaring out of my clock radio, furious at myself for "not being strong enough" the night before. "No one wants to be defeated" so I'd restrict again, punishing myself with even fewer crackers and half an apple for lunch. But night would fall, and the ice cream would call. This would repeat all week long until Friday arrived, and it was time to celebrate getting through the week. We all need a "cheat day," right?

Burned out from a week of binging and restricting, by the time I got that first greasy slice in my mouth, I couldn't stop. Once, while complaining about my weight to one of my mom's skinny friends at our favorite pizza joint, she had the audacity to suggest I only eat one piece of pizza. As if! Her words lingered in the air and left a deeply troubling feeling that something was desperately wrong with me. I immediately shoved the troubling feeling down with iceberg lettuce smothered in ranch dressing. At least I didn't dip the pizza in ranch, right?

That conversation haunts me to this day whenever I eat more than one piece of pizza. It was not possible for me to eat only one piece then … and wouldn't be for at least thirty more years. Even now, I approach pizza with extreme caution.

My dad took me running and cycling. We conquered a bike trip together with my youth group from Santa Cruz to San Luis Obispo. I was obsessed with how fat my knees looked in bike shorts. I loved being with my dad and hated the photos. My mom taught me about fat-free food swaps. She crafted delicious meals from scratch and managed her portions with the self-discipline of a five-star general. I tried to follow her example, but the piles of food I ate to survive final exams, mean girls, and school dances were not something any amount of swapping, biking, or jazzercise could shed. I wish I knew then what I know now—that you can't out-grapevine a bad diet.

My perfectly organized extreme eating plan swinging from high-fat binges to fat-free fixes took its toll as fear of weight gain controlled me. Food was my obsession, and the scale was my guide. Turns out, whatever the scale said gave me permission to eat. Didn't lose weight? What's the point … eat! Lost weight? Great! Eat! Food, fear, and the number on the scale tangled into a mental mess. The only way to not be afraid of gaining weight was to restrict, and the only way to not be afraid of experiencing all the uncomfortable feelings was to eat all the food.

I remember one day, before my senior year of high school, our youth group had an end-of-the-summer barbecue. I dieted hard and finally reached my goal weight—155. I missed swimsuit season, but I was thin, and that meant I could gorge without guilt. Thanks to my inability to resist a creamy church casserole, or three, it was the last and only time I saw 155 pop up on the bathroom scale.

And then I stopped growing.

The Freshman 40
1990: 18 Years Old

With Wilson Phillips in my ears and the groove in my heart—I was off to college. Oh, glorious day! After unloading half the house on the lawn in front of the dorm, my parents hit the road with one less child, my brother waving from the back seat. I jumped for joy and skedaddled to the cafeteria for orientation. Ah, the sweet smell of baked goods, powdered bleach, and hormones. It was there, surrounded by the clamor of newly minted college kids just released into the wild, that I met new friends, new authorities, and the local soft-serve machine. When we were excused, I grabbed five cookies to go, in case my roommate wanted one, and trotted off to the all-girls floor that would be my home away from parents for the next year. Somebody pinch me (and here's hoping he looks like Keanu).

I loved college, my new friends, my new church, and riding my bike across town to grab frozen yogurt. I was not prepared for all the new emotions that came with every new experience, especially being rejected by college boys.

The early 1990's pressure to have a boy like you because it confirmed your social status as "wife material" was not a social norm I was mature enough to process. A cute boy might ignore me, but food never rejected me, was always up for a good time, and made me feel secure when I was lonely. Goooooo snickerdoodles!

The Bible says there is a way that seems right to a person that, in the end, only leads to death (Proverbs 14:12). It felt right to eat when I felt wrong. Bad grade? Food cheered me. Feeling invisible in a class of 400? Food was comforting. Can't fit into my pants? Food distracted me. Food became friend, fortifier, fixer, *and* the catalyst of deep-seated suffering. As I stepped on the scale, shattering all personal records week after week, I had no idea how to stop the freight train of food as it mowed through my life, leaving wreckage in the wake.

I ate and gained, ate, and gained. When I wasn't studying, skipping class—oh, I mean going to class—or napping, I was foraging for food.

Eating was my activity of choice. Eating was my hobby, my source of energy, and my sense of accomplishment. If I could finish nothing else, I could finish a plate of food. Go me! I was putting so much pressure on food to be the solution that it had become the problem.

I grew more despondent and desperate to be loved by others because I hated myself every time I saw my reflection, put on pants, or breathed. I just knew I would be happier if I pleased my friends, if I pleased my parents, and if I pleased my professors. I could not please all the people all the time, so I'd switch gears and please myself with food. What I didn't recognize at the time is that pleasing people *is* rewarding, but it isn't guaranteed. Food was guaranteed to please me, but that reward system was morphing into addiction faster than I could say "pass the creamsicles."

Bottom line: Food was winning the dopamine reward pleasure war while torpedoing my self-esteem. Momentary "innocent" pleasure was causing me catastrophic agony that would devastate me for decades. The hollowness in my soul would not be filled with food no matter how valiant my effort. I needed a work-around fast. How could I **know** I was deeply loved and valued even if I was desperately empty and overweight?

A boyfriend. That should do it. Finding a boy who loved me for the size of my heart, not my booty … I mean body… would solve everything.

(*radio static* "Alert! Alert! Mayday! Mayday!" *radio static*)
Did you hear something? Shrug. Pass the tuna casserole.

I'd like to pause here and identify a common thought pattern that fueled my eating. It went something like this:

If I just had _____, I would be happy (more time, weight loss, a boyfriend, good grades, a car that worked), and if I didn't have any one of those things, carrot cake would suffice. But I had to have all of them to be happy. The truth about life is that there's always a "happiness void." If we use unhappiness as an excuse to eat, there will always be a reason to eat.

Pursuing happiness in the form of pleasure is fleeting and ultimately damaging as a way of life. But my ability to understand life and food and God was more mixed up than a half-eaten box of Nuts and Nougats after a train wreck. To prove it, I concluded that if I was loved by a boy who loved me for who I was inside, the outside wouldn't matter. If the outside didn't matter, I could continue eating *and* feel loved. Problem solved.

I incorrectly believed that if I was loved, it meant I was good. The opposite was also true—if I wasn't loved, it meant I was bad. I felt overweight and unworthy of love, and as a result, I confused the "feel good" feeling food provided with the "worthiness" I really needed that only comes from the Lord.

"But God shows his great love for us in that while we were still sinners Christ died for us." (Romans 5:8 ESV)

Clueless and hoodwinked by momentary pleasure, I simultaneously (1) filled up on food to feel right and (2) suffered the consequences of gluttony that made my whole self feel wrong.

This line of thinking spiraled into an inner turmoil that went something like this: eating made me feel good but eating like I did was bad; therefore, I deserved to be disgusting. I was a horrible person for eating; thankfully, I could eat to feel better. Junk food makes me feel gross, but that's what I get for eating it. I'm such a loser; let's have a pie.

Enter: self-loathing with a side of shame.

Self-loathing is the desolate destination of those of us who pull our self-worth from anything other than our Father in Heaven.

I believed at the time that a boyfriend and lots of delicious food would make me feel better.

What I really needed was to go to God, not food or people, to fix my hurting heart.

1 Peter 5:7 says:
"Give all your worries to Him because He cares for you." (NLV)
I knew this verse, but I didn't know how to go to God with my "little food problem." How could He possibly care about something so trivial? He had bigger pancakes to flip, and I had other things I'd rather involve Him in, like how to pass Statistics. When it came to the proverbial house of my life, God could enter any room He wanted—except the kitchen. But why would He want to come in there? Don't make me laugh. God doesn't eat anyway.

But there was a fire blazing in my kitchen that threatened to flatten my entire house, and He was the only one with a working fire extinguisher.

Now Showing: "Nuts and Nougats Goes on a Manhunt."

Have your popcorn ready.

Without the connection between God and food, I looked for approval from college boys because that was the only way I could prove to myself I was a desirable human being regardless of my weight.

I *was* valuable, but I didn't *feel* valuable because I didn't weigh 155. I shared my desire to have a boyfriend with trusted people in my life. One person told me boys only took an interest in thin girls, so for a boy to see past my figure to my personality was unlikely. Another told me there were so many thin girls out there that, statistically, I didn't stand a chance. Another said no boy would ever love me if I was fat. Gee, thanks, that was helpful. I was living a nightmare of cycling shame, and circumstances were confirming my self-hate.

Did I mention that my roommate had a steady boyfriend *and* could eat peanut butter and whipped honey sandwiches without gaining an ounce? My jealousy festered like maggots in my despairing heart.

To give you an idea of how messed up I was, she loved the Lord and was my friend (not like the friends with the great fat girl advice mentioned above). On the contrary, she was a kind, compassionate, and playful person. We met at Leadership Training Camp the summer before freshman year and freaked when we realized we were attending the same college. Before camp ended, we prayed that we would live close together and see each other often.

When I got my roommate placement letter in the mail, I tore it open. Her name was listed as my roommate.

Just to clarify: We never requested each other because we met too late in the summer for that. She requested a morning person as a roommate. I asked for a night person. She asked for a suite; I checked the box for the all-girls floor. We were headed to different complexes until the Lord stepped in and placed us in the same room on the all-girls floor, just us, together.

She was a blessing to me, but her boyfriend was so annoying, constantly spoiling her with sweet notes, date nights, and flowers. Our room had bike hooks on the ceiling to save floor space. But for some reason, we never hung our bikes on the hooks. What we did hang on the hooks were all the flippin' flowers he gave her. She dried them and rotated them weekly. The hooks were always filled with gorgeous upside-down bouquets specially picked just for her. Gag me. (See me lying on my bed, falling asleep every night looking up. No wonder I had nightmares.)

One boy captured my attention. He was a tall glass of Eric Stoltz with a spikey sprig of Dennis Leary—but my crush on him was no joke. Insecure about my physical appearance, I still tried to get his attention. Was it too much? He didn't notice me anyway, but I told myself, "What do you expect being so fat?" One day I bopped into the common room and saw him sitting and chatting with a petite, pretty girl I'd never seen before. I smiled, and he introduced me, saying, "This is Julia. She's nothing."

I was fat, I was nothing, and I was devastated.

Around that time, I was feeling extra heavy, which ballooned my self-loathing and shame. I remember trying to sleep and covering my eyes with my pillow to block the view of the hanging flowers. One night, I raged at God and cried out, "Haven't I been good to you, God? Haven't I done what you've asked me and obeyed you and served you since I was five? Why can't you do this for me? Why can't you provide someone to love me?"

It's a wonder I didn't get a boyfriend in the shape of a lightning bolt to the head. Arrogant, angry, and broken, the jealousy stirred up by those stupid flowers rotted me from the inside out.

"I've got it!" I declared in a silent prayer, "Lord, there is an empty bike hook for once. Please show me that you have someone for me by giving me flowers to dry on that hook. Please." And I fell asleep on a tear-drenched, snot-soaked pillow facing the wall.

A couple of nights later, I was alone in our dorm room late at night. To give you the lay of the land, we were on the second level on an all-girls floor. Stairs leading to the first floor were across from our door to the right. At the bottom of the stairs were the first-floor hallway and a heavy exit door. After a certain hour, all the doors were locked, and you couldn't get in unless you had a key. I was alone in the room; it was around midnight, and I was rummaging in the cupboards above our closet.

Suddenly, there was a knock on our door. Strange. Had my roommate left her key? Did my best friend Julie need to borrow a protractor?

I opened the door.

In front of me stood a young man, and in his outstretched hand was a single red long-stemmed rose. My eyes fixed on the beautiful flower as my prayer of desperation flashed through my mind. Could it possibly be?

"Would you like a rose?" he asked. I reached for the rose, took it in my fingers, and brought my head up to thank him—*but he was gone*. I looked up and down the hallway; I ran down the stairs and through the downstairs hall, spinning, my eyes darting everywhere. No person, not a one—anywhere. No doors opening. No doors slamming shut, no talking. Silence. Stillness. The young man was gone.

The Lord answered my prayer. I believe it was an angel sent from the Lord to deliver me a rose. A single flower that we understand represents love. Special delivery from His heart to mine. Like the woman at the well, He saw me. He heard me and responded to me with what I *really* needed—to be seen, understood, and deeply loved.

Everything was going to be ok.

I hung that rose on the empty bike hook. I dried it, and today it sits in a box with a note my beloved husband had the best man hand deliver to me on our wedding day … "Meet me at the altar at 6:00. I'll be waiting."

My obsession to land a boy left me, but the obsession with food did not.

I'd arrive home that summer carrying forty extra pounds and would wrestle with my weight until I graduated with a bachelor's degree in Yo-Yo Dieting Summa Cum Laude.

Love Walked In
1995: 23 Years Old

After college, I completed a summer internship at Levi Strauss and Company. Originally, I meant to spend the summer working at a Christian camp with a dear friend I'd palled around with since middle school. I couldn't pass up the opportunity to make acid-washed jeans, so he headed to the Santa Cruz mountains without me. When it was all over, we'd meet up for Christian Music Day at Paramount's Great America and catch up.

The end of August arrived, we finalized the plans, and he told me he was bringing a friend he met at camp. Great. That boy had more dates than a desk calendar. Fine. Eye roll.

As for me, I was recovering from an on-again-off-again relationship that saw its final demise when he tossed me into some bushes for leaning against his freshly waxed CHP magnet. "Don't ever do that again," he growled. "I won't," I promised and never contacted him again.

At the amusement park waiting in line for the Top Gun ride, I spotted my friend and his friend walking toward us through the crowd. To my surprise, he was not with a girl. Instead, he was walking next to the most gorgeous guy I'd ever seen.

A head above the swirling mass of people, The Most Gorgeous Guy I'd Ever Seen cut a line straight for me through the crowd. As we stood face to face and reached out to shake hands, my brother says he could "see the sparks fly off us."

Craig, at twenty-one, already owned and operated his own video production business. He had hair like Dean Forester and a smile like Maverick … take my breath away. He loved rock climbing, skydiving, and Jesus. He was joyful, fun, kind, and confident. Kick the tires and light the fires.

A zit on my chin the size of Kilimanjaro made seeing my actual face a challenge. Also, I was nowhere near my goal weight, and I thought John Lennon sunglasses were cool. Yet, he stayed close, and we talked to each other all day long.

The stars came out, and we all went back to Craig's house to watch the highly acclaimed romantic movie: ALIENS. Sitting next to each other on a very small couch, it was all we could do not to hold hands. Terrified by our immediate and consuming attraction, I ran out the door as the credits rolled and waited in a dark driveway while the others said goodbye. This perfect young man seemed to be interested in me, but I must have misunderstood. This is me we're talking about. Pig Legs. Nothing. The girl with a colossal blemish who just got tossed into some bushes because she was less important than a buff job on a mediocre muscle car. I needed to disappear fast before I got my hopes up. Why were they taking so long?

The next day, after a good night's sleep, I had a clear head to think logically. I had spent less than 24 hours with the guy, and I needed to be rational. So, I did what any girl would do. I called my best friend Julie and told her that I had met the man I was going to marry yesterday but had no way to contact him because I took to the street faster than Jackie Joyner-Kersee with a new pair of sneakers. She laughed and promised to pray for me. We caught up on life, I reminded her to pray for me, she promised again, and we hung up.

Meanwhile, Craig was calling me, hitting redial, getting a busy signal, and calling again. For those of you who are too young to remember "call waiting," it was when society finally had the technology to put one call on hold and take another call from a landline. It cost extra, and we didn't have it. Craig had to dial, hear a busy signal, hang up, and dial again. Kind of like punching a vending machine hoping the chips will fall.

When I finally hung up the phone, it immediately rang. "Hello?" Craig's upbeat voice greeted me and asked if I'd like to go out with him *on a date* to San Francisco. It took a millisecond to check my calendar. Turns out my schedule was wide open.

He took me to Planet Hollywood in San Francisco and did a magic trick with a saltshaker. He took me to Vista Point overlooking the Golden Gate Bridge and did a magic trick with my heart.

Two days later, at the beach on the steps of a lifeguard hut, he told me he wanted "an exclusive relationship and to work toward something permanent."

Two years later, at my home church, we swapped rings and spit in front of hundreds of people, grinning ear to ear and pledging to love each other forever.

… and he never even saw me at my goal weight.

An Entrepreneur on Endless Diets
2004: Age 32

We spent our newlywed year in Sunnyvale, then hitched a U-Haul to our rusty Ford Explorer, jostling all the way down to Los Angeles. Craig would live his dream to break into the movie business, and I would take the fashion industry by storm … and find the best Huevos Rancheros in West LA. On a quiet Sunday, we were swindled into the perfect apartment—a hovel on a firetruck route with black mold behind our bedpost, termite eggs in our bathroom, and Nakatomi Tower right outside our living room window. Yippee-ki-yay … we made the big time, baby!

While Craig and his camera helped Buffy slay vampires, I designed accessories and clothing for several sportswear companies until we went to Prague where he was a camera operator on Blade 2 for six months. I took a leave of absence from work and joined him, and Prague became my hometown. Dragging broken bags of groceries from Tesco over cobblestone streets in the rain, learning a formidable language in a medieval city, and almost getting kidnapped by Gypsies turned me into a round peg that didn't fit into a cubicle anymore. I quit my job and set out to make my own way in fashion.

Before long, it was 2004, the thong song was ringing in our ears, Napoleon Dynamite brought tater tots back, and Benifer split for the first time. I paired my desire to fight cancer with my middle school sense of humor, and voilà, Ta-tas® Brand Clothing and the Save the Ta-tas® foundation were born. The brand shocked and delighted Fred Segal customers across Santa Monica and soon the country. Once Kate Beckinsale was seen in Us Weekly wearing one of my shirts coming out of her trailer, we couldn't make the tanks and tees fast enough. I was living my dream in LA—happily married, attending a wonderful church, and running a booming charitable business that inspired joy in the face of disastrous diagnoses. These were the years we funded amazing research; I was named a most influential woman by Transworld Business and presented with a humanitarian award.

I struggled to keep up with the totally realistic LA size 0 beauty aesthetic despite being obsessed with food. Radio interviews with shock jocks at 4 a.m. were a blast, but TV spots were terrifying. I couldn't find anything to wear (even though I had a clothing line), dreaded being on camera, and couldn't look at myself in photos.

One day, I arrived in Culver City, CA, to be interviewed on a popular talk show hosted by a gorgeous woman. Cresting over 200 pounds, I searched for weeks for a shirt I felt ok wearing on camera. The crew was panicking because the tiny polka dot optics on the blouse I bought were ruining the shot. One of the producers, desperate to fix my wardrobe malfunction, let me borrow her leather jacket. She was a size 4. I went on stage and did the spot … but for all the negative self-talk and self-body shaming swirling in my head, you'd think I was performing a version of *"Fat Girl In Little Coat"* that would have made Chris Farley and the entire cast of *Tommy Boy* proud. I was so embarrassed by my physical appearance I barely remember the experience. Luckily, I have the pictures to prove I was there, and come to think of it, pictures to prove I once wore a size 4.

I tried every new-fangled diet I found. Weight Watchers no longer worked for me. Body for Life got me below 160. Nutrisystem didn't suit my taste. Lindora got me to 158 the first round, but not the five times after, and I never reached my goal weight. I left each program with the sign of an "L" on my forehead to quote Smash Mouth. Hopelessness crept in and took root.

And then we decided to have kids.

Motherhood …

Why Is Everything So Sticky?
2008: 36 years old

I forgot to tell you that on an October day in 1989, during a game of pool at youth group, I discerned God telling me I would not birth children but adopt. I agreed and racked for a break when the Loma Prieta earthquake slammed our community. Ducking under the table as my world jolted, I knew in my heart that God had a plan for my life, that it was good, and that my children would be adopted.

One other person I forgot to mention this to was Craig. Uh oh. Imagine my surprise when he thought starting a family meant I would birth our children myself. Did he have a screw loose? Hold your horses, cowboy … God *said* I was going to adopt my kids.

Unfortunately, God had not told Craig yet.

How had I left out this teeny tiny cosmic detail in all our deep, heartfelt conversations? His eyes. Clearly, I had been distracted by Craig's blue eyes and completely forgot to mention our adopted children for years. Rookie move!

Confused and sad, I asked God to tell Craig the plan sometime soon. Until then, I decided to give getting pregnant the old college try. We removed the goalie, prayed … and well, you get the idea.

Years went by, and not once did we see the faintest double line on that plastic bad news stick.

I didn't mention adoption again. Was it my imagination that God told me I was going to adopt? I knew the Lord had a plan for my life, and I trusted Him with it. If He said it, He would make a way; if He didn't, that would become clear too.

"Be still and know that I am God." (Psalm 46:10 NIV)

On a date night in October of 2008, while swishing wasabi into soy sauce waiting for Kanpachi, Craig said out of the blue, "Let's adopt."

I had the agency on speed dial, and within a matter of days, we were sitting smack dab in the back of an orientation meeting on the edge of our seats, ready to bolt if it got too hot. We almost left after the administration portion, stayed for the interviews, and hauled home a stack of paperwork that paired nicely with a couple of cases of Red Vines. Within two weeks, we were drilling magnetic locks into our kitchen cupboards and on track to be the fastest couple to complete the certification process in our region. Not that we're competitive.

There are a jillion considerations and zillion decisions during the process of adoption.

We had four simple requests of God:

1. Fast.
2. Easy legal.
3. Twins.
4. Healthy.

The agency told us we should be happy to have one child within a year because the process takes time, and twins are rarely placed for adoption. Two weeks into our fost/adopt certification (although we didn't know it at the time), our twins were born. Two months later, three business days after our paperwork was finalized (and on the first day of demolition to build a bathroom for the nursery), we received a call that we had been chosen to be the parents of twin girls born at home. They were waiting for us in a nearby hospital. We jumped up and down in our front yard, stared with horrified faces at the drywall on the side of the house, and raced to the hospital.

Arriving at the pediatrics wing, we were shuffled into the tiny nursing mothers' room next to the NICU. It was packed with two doctors, three nurses, two social workers, the head of the department, and child protective services, arms crossed and glaring at us from the corner. Two empty chairs sat in the center of the crowd, one for each of us. That's not awkward. We clutched hands as the story unfolded.

Two months ago, 911 received a call that twins were born at home. The tiny twins were 26 1/2 weeks, frozen blue, and near dead. Baby A was barely breathing. Baby B had a stage 3 brain bleed.

The prognosis was not good, but they survived.

Because their birth mother was unable to care for them, and their closest relative lived far away, Baby A and Baby B had been nurtured only by rotating NICU nurses. God bless those nurses!

Current status? Both had severe muscle tone issues, torticollis, and possible holes in their hearts typical of preemies. Baby B was still heavily medicated to prevent seizures. Words like "cerebral palsy," "wheelchairs," and "brain damage" clanged in our ears as each member of the staff gave us their professional opinion.

"We can't know what happened in the house when they were born."
"You don't have to do this."
"You can't see them unless you decide to adopt them. They are not puppies."
"We understand if you need to go home and think about it."

Silence fell over the room. It was our turn to speak.

"Are they healthy now?" My husband asked.
"Yes," the doctors nodded. The seizure medication was preventative, and aside from muscle tone issues and a small footnote that they hadn't taken a bottle yet, everything "seemed fine."

"What is the legal situation with their birth family?" I asked
"All settled," replied the social worker.

The crowd flooded out of the room, the door shut, and we faced each other in complete agreement. The Lord had answered our prayers.

1. Fast √
2. Easy legal √
3. Twins √
4. Healthy today √ (That's all we can ever ask. Who knows what will happen tomorrow?)

We laughed and embraced and scrubbed up to meet our new daughters. They were beautiful.

There was just one teeny tiny cloud on the horizon.

Both refused to eat.

Feeding "The Unfeedable"

We teamed up with nurses and therapists to help the girls latch onto a bottle. Their gag reflex was on their lips instead of their tonsil area, so whenever their lips touched anything, they would projectile vomit. The hospital would not discharge them unless they ate, but they couldn't, and there was no explanation as to why not.

They needed specialized heart monitoring, brain tests, and to see a deformity specialist. The best-case recovery scenario required early intervention, and time was ticking. Physical therapy, occupational therapy, and developmental therapy all should have started at home yesterday. When their due date came and went, we made the difficult decision to surgically insert ports in their tummies through which we poured formula until that day (Lord willing) they could eat and drink orally.

After the surgery took place, we wrapped our two bundles in ducky onesies and said goodbye to the NICU. The firemen who brought them to the hospital that fateful night over three months earlier surprised us with a visit, held the girls one last time, and double-checked the car seats.

At home, the real rehab began. My husband built specialized bouncy seats that allowed us to tube feed two babies at one time. Craig and I would teach our girls to eat, talk, walk, and achieve their personal best outcome, and we knew we couldn't get there alone. The Lord provided us with a dream team to help, and we are eternally grateful to all the specialists who assisted amidst endless setbacks.

Therapists descended on our home almost every day. Social workers checked in. We were up most of the night feeding. RSV was spreading fast, and the respiratory doctor demanded we isolate because their lungs would not survive infection. Babysitters were out of the question.

One challenge we didn't expect: aspiration. This means the girls would suck fluid into their lungs while they were spitting up and trying to breathe at the same time. Feeding required knowing how to clear their lungs and save their life at any time.

They vomited all day long. We had painter's plastic on the carpet, puke on the ceiling, and changed their clothes 9 to 12 times a day.

I'm still a pro at catching vomit in my shirt #winning.

Desperate for respite, I posted an ad on a local NICU corkboard for a home nurse to come so we could sleep or get groceries. The nurse who answered the call stayed with us for three years. She was as sweet, gentle, and kind as Cinderella's fairy godmother, and Craig says if she didn't cash our checks, he would have thought she was an angel. She was a godsend.

What does this have to do with my food story? I'm glad you asked…

For the next two years, everything in our life revolved around food. Our twins had been labeled "The Unfeedable" in county documents, therefore our number one priority was to to help our daughters beat the odds, eat and gain weight.

We had the best OT, PT, and developmental therapists this side of heaven teaching our daughters to eat the fattiest, most delicious foods we could find. Ice cream, whipped cream, hummus, bananas, avocados… if it had a high-carb, high-fat content, we were enticing them to eat it. The occupational therapist came each week and requested I fill the fridge with every fattening food she could think of. She had me buy things like whipped cream, nut butters, chocolate sauce, and honey for them to practice touching and tasting just in case that food became the food that transitioned them to eating solids.

But they didn't eat all that food. Guess who did? Not my husband … not the dog …

In this season of survival, at home all day with an endless supply of fatty food while feeling broken-down, inadequate, frustrated, weary, isolated, and scared - food was an ever-present comfort, and my obsession with food spiraled.

Prayers were constantly flowing from my lips. In fact, one night when they were eleven months, one girl wasn't crawling, neither was eating, and everything was soaked in vomit. I wept and begged the Lord, "Please help me! PLEASE HEAL THEM!" I believed He loved us, and He would help.

Nevertheless the process took time. It was all so overwhelming that food soothed me in a second like nothing else. I see now, I trusted God with the future, but food made the moment manageable. Unfortunately, what I didn't see was that trusting food in the moment made the future unbearable and robbed God of the opportunity to help me both in the moment *and* in the future. Food was soothing me, then smothering me, and I was suffocating under an avalanche of cheesy pasta and cookie dough.

It was early December (three months later) when Craig proposed adding a wheelchair ramp to our front porch for our twin who was still not crawling. She was 14 months old and could only sit. Then, right before Christmas, I watched her (in one move) lie down, roll over, get on her hands and knees, and crawl. Just like that, she was trailing after the dog, escaping her sister, and giggling as she glided across the painter's plastic. It was a Christmas miracle. Soon, she watched Craig eat a banana and licked her lips. Craig asked her if she wanted some, and she nodded. He gave her a taste, and she didn't throw up. Her sister couldn't allow a tasty banana be enjoyed without her, and before long, both girls were eating bananas and cookies. Mostly cookies.

At our next appointment, I told the doctor that they were eating, but they only wanted cookies.
"How many a day?" He asked
"Eight … or so," I hedged.
"Julia," he chuckled, "I know it's exciting that they are eating, but I think they are taking advantage. Let's get that number down."

As the girls and I added veggies to our diet, their willingness to try new foods slowly expanded. They were two and a half years old the day we finally spread blankets on the kitchen floor, kissed their rosy cheeks, praised the Lord, prayed like crazy, *removed the g-tubes*, and never looked back.

I was the heaviest I had ever been.

How Did I Get Here?
My First Visit to an Addiction Program

I'm not sure how I ended up at the dingy door of a Van Nuys food addiction program. I do remember sitting outside talking myself out of going in when the song "Healing Begins" by Tenth Avenue North came on the radio. I took the lyrics as a sign, locked the car twice, and entered the rooms for the first time.

Surrounded by wood paneling, burnt coffee smell, and depressed people made focusing difficult. The two men behind me discussing where to get burritos after made me doubt the effectiveness of the program. The leader expected me to tell everyone my name and that I was a "compulsive overeater" … out loud. Good luck with that. I attended half-heartedly for a few weeks, lost a few pounds, and ditched the rooms faster than Road Runner escaping a barrel of TNT.

Thank goodness that was over.

In less than a month, I gained it all back and more.

Did I Turn Off the Toaster?
2010: 38 years old.

I raced through my days, dividing time between family, two businesses, and church. Anxiety rattled me to the core. One fall day at a harvest fair petting zoo with the girls, fear so gripped me that I visited a counselor soon after. Sitting across from her, I listed all the reasons baby animals and bouncy slides ignited panic in my brain, needing her to tell me I was "normal."

She sent me to a psychiatrist.
That escalated quickly.

Telling no one, I donned an oversized sun hat and dark glasses and jumped in and out of shadows all the way to his office. He opened the door and asked me if I was in witness protection. Then he listened to my story.

When I stopped talking, he shuffled through his desk files and handed me a sheet of paper that looked like he'd copied it many times over many years for many people.

"Do you ever experience any of this?" he asked.

It was a list of feelings, thoughts, and fears. Some I couldn't relate to, but others broke me. I couldn't believe the hidden pain I'd tried to handle myself for decades was described in black and white, right on that very sheet he'd been sharing with people for years. Why hadn't I told someone sooner?

I started sobbing, totally fogging up my sunglasses.

"Yes," I replied, "since I was 7."

He diagnosed me with OCD on the spot.

Specifically, I was afraid of germs, had a checking disorder (meaning I felt the need to check the garage door, front door, curling iron, toaster, oven, and/or the stovetop several times before leaving the house) and a form of what I like to call "shoe-drop-o-phobia," meaning I often had anxiety something horrible would happen. I had a secret internal name for these thoughts. I called them "daymares," like nightmares only they tortured my mind in broad daylight while doing daily activities like driving or cooking.

He told me OCD is like Tourette's. You can't help that these things just pop up and cycle through your mind over and over incessantly. It's chemical and could be treated with medication. It wasn't my fault, it was time for meds, and I could no longer handle it myself. I agreed to abide by the prescription for the sake of healing.

Between us, this was very difficult for me. I didn't want to have OCD, and I didn't want to take meds. He explained that if I had a torn meniscus, of course, I would treat it. How was a brain that didn't produce enough serotonin any different? He assured me that OCD can be cured with behavior modification in time and a small dose of medication for now. So began the long road of facing my fears, modifying behavior, and managing medication.

I was diagnosed the day after we took out the g-tubes.

Looking back, I believe God used my OCD for good—He used my fear of germs to help me protect the girls from RSV. He used my need to check everything multiple times to allow me to give them accurate medicine doses and proper care. He used someone like me, so afraid of something bad happening, to protect them from real dangers that others might not notice. He used me, flaws and all, to help two little babies learn how to eat, walk, talk, and enjoy the world. But now it was time for me to heal.

The effects of Fluoxetine astonished me. I couldn't believe that "normal" people's brains felt like this, so calm and content. I practiced behavior modification, stopped worrying about the curling iron, felt great and gained 50 pounds.

What 220 Feels Like

Recovering from OCD became my priority. I was gaining weight fast, but the doctor told me Fluoxetine does not cause weight gain. He said I was just eating too much and didn't realize it.

It was a season of rapid-fire diets. I'd go on a very strict meal plan from the time I woke up until noon. Nothing worked past one o'clock in the afternoon. By 4:30 I had a sugary latte in one hand and pre-dinner snacks in the other. Dinner with the kids at 5:00, another dinner when my husband got home around 8:00, and more food goodies at 9:30 while we watched American Idol.

Years went by. By the time I was diagnosed with fatty liver, I was so large I couldn't reach my shoes to tie them. Lucky for me, I *could* reach the chocolate hidden on top of the fridge, which always made me feel better about my weight.

Filled with self-loathing and no longer fitting into my largest pair of jeans, I went to my doctor and asked for the sleeve, a form of gastrectomy where the doctor laparoscopically staples closed the larger, curved part of the stomach. It was offered to patients who were obese, and I was obese. I came packed and ready for same-day surgery with her green light.

She pressed a clipboard to her chest and adjusted her glasses.

"Julia," she sighed, "you don't have any comorbid conditions. I can't do this for you. What you need is a 12-step program."

One of my nonexistent comorbid conditions flared up and almost killed me on the spot. No! I was NOT going back to that dingy office in Van Nuys with the "let's go binge on burritos after" gang. I already did the 12-steps, and they didn't work.

She waited for a response.

"OK," I mumbled,

"Promise me you'll go to 30 meetings in 30 days?" She tapped her pen.

ARE YOU INSANE, DOCTOR LADY???

"OK," I repeated. Waddling out of the room, I conspired to return for my surgery as soon as the 12-steps failed, just like they did before.

A Prophetic Word from a Friend

It was about this time I got a call from a dear friend who said God "put me on her heart," and gave her a vision about me. She asked if she could share.

Spoiler alert—prophetic visions freaked me out. Here's why: long ago in a galaxy far, far away, at high school youth group, a visiting pastor came to our meeting and started speaking over the group, saying things like, "Someone here is being influenced by sexual sin," then scanned for guilty faces and pointing. We were high schoolers. Like, who wasn't under their covers with a flashlight reading romance novels after the parents went to bed? So, nope. I did not want to hear her vision.

"Sure." Was my nose growing?

Apparently, while she was praying for me, she saw a t-shaped handle lodged in my skull, sticking out of my head, and the spiritual forces of evil were using it to control me.

That's horrifying. Internal screaming.

"Thank you." I said calmly, "I'll pray about it." I couldn't hang up fast enough.

I knew, in the way you know deep in your knower …

The "handle" was *food*.

Food had a handle on me, alright, and now I had a mental picture of what was really going on in my spiritual life as it related to my eating. Healing would take time and be painful and removing the "handle" would leave a "hole in my head" only the Holy Spirit could fill. I knew that the Lord had a plan for my life; He was with me, and He would fix me, so I prayed.

I asked God to remove the "handle."
I asked God to fill the void with His Spirit alone.
I asked God to forgive my sin and help me repent.
I asked God to release me from bondage.

A vision came to me of the Lord removing the handle completely, filling the hole in my head with His Spirit like healing oil or salve, bandaging and tending to the wound.

He also gave me a gentle word of warning: choose not to put the handle back. For this, I was going to need His help every moment of every day.

The First Step Take Two
2015: 43 years old

I still needed to keep the promise I made to my doctor. But an addict?? ME??? Not possible. I am a CHRISTIAN! Christians aren't addicts! We have JESUS!! I wrestled with going into "the rooms" again (which is what 12-steppers call the confidential rooms where we meet with fellow addicts in recovery).

My husband had a very busy schedule working on a TV show, but he was home in the early mornings for the next month, so as providence would have it, I could go to 30 meetings in 30 days at 6 a.m. UGH. 6 a.m., really? Maybe no one would be there, and the meeting would be canceled. Maybe I could sit in the back, and no one would see me. If I just did what the doctor prescribed and it didn't work, surely, she'd agree to bariatric surgery.

I woke up at 5 a.m., squeezed into some stretchy black pants with the size tag ripped out, and drove to the run-down, atrium-style building. It was cold, quiet, with a layer of mist that hung like a shroud in the center. I pressed a button on the elevator that dinged throughout the foggy, open air.

Down a dim hallway, I found the marked door to the meeting and reminded myself of the goal. "Just do your time to get the green light for surgery." I condemned myself for being so fat I had to come to this horrible place. "Just sit in the back and don't talk to anyone. You got this, girl!" I breathed deep and turned the handle.

"The Revenant" is a term that means "a person who returns from the dead." In theaters, Leo DiCaprio plays Hugh Glass, a man mauled by a bear. Nearly dead, after cauterizing his own wounds, he drags himself to another human in the middle of nowhere for help. I would later compare myself to The Revenant that day. Dragging myself into a meeting, mauled by the bear of food, and after failing to fix my wounds, I went in search of someone to help me survive.

There she was, sitting alone in the front, looking right at me. No escape, no sitting in the back. We were the only two people in the room. I was late and she was talking … to me.

"Welcome!" she announced. "I'm so glad you're here; I can't have a meeting by myself."

Perfect. Just great. I smiled. "Good to be here!" Yah, no.

As I sat across from her, a few others trickled in. She connected me with two women, and we all went to coffee after. One of them agreed to be my sponsor on the spot.

She was kind but firm and let me talk about my struggles. She had bariatric surgery, and it didn't go well. She was a good friend and resource, but God was my main "sponsor". I didn't want to replace one idol (food) for another idol (a person). Now was the time for me to see idols fail, learn from my mistakes, and lean on the Lord alone.

"Trust the Lord with all your heart and lean not on your own understanding. In all your ways acknowledge Him, and He will direct your path." (Proverbs 3:5)

Three Steps Forward

At the beginning of the program, my anger boiled because I couldn't eat "like other people" and be thin. It took time to process this resentment. They say in program, "It takes the time it takes," so I did my best to settle in for a long journey with the Lord, good days and the hangry too. The first year in program I worked on the first three steps only.

1. I admitted I was powerless over food.
2. I came to believe that a power greater than myself could restore me to sanity.
3. I made a decision to turn my will and my life over to the care of God as I understood Him.
   -The Big Book of Alcoholics Anonymous

If you're a Christian and you love Jesus, you might feel a little uncomfortable with these vague references to an unidentified "higher power." Welcome to program where everyone chooses their own god, but I was not allowed to share what I knew about the saving power of Jesus Christ alone, Elohim, The One True God. As a result, I never felt at home in the rooms.

This is the crux of the issue. There was a man named Jesus who lived on earth, did many miracles, and claimed to be the Messiah. He was hated for that claim, as well as the loving miracles He did, by many in the religious and political establishment. He was arrested and endured an illegal trial held in the middle of the night. Next, brutally beaten and nailed to a cross, He would hang publically with criminals, as a criminal even though He did nothing wrong. Then He died, and the earth shook. Three days later, He rose from the dead, and His resurrection power was so mighty, others were raised with Him, all of this witnessed by many people in the city which is a recorded historical fact. You can read the testimonies of eyewitnesses in the Bible text, but it is confirmed elsewhere. The crucifixion and resurrection of Jesus of Nazareth set Him apart as THE POWER. The only Higher Power that can save us. There isn't another God, and He proved it by his life, death and resurrection - and work in our lives today.

I've done a lot of research on the Gospels because I am, by nature, a skeptic. I trust… and do my homework. The Christian faith is backed by reliable history and modern day experience. Every human needs to examine the historical documents of the resurrection and decide what to do with the historical records and phenomenon that is Jesus.

It's clear to me Jesus is God. The ONLY God. No other has done what He did and does what He does. Therefore, it breaks my heart when people pray to created things like dead people, ravens, wolves, or even themselves because these types of higher powers are false gods and can't save us.

So, when I was asked to choose the prayer, I chose "The Lord's Prayer." When I was allowed to name my Higher Power, I used the name of Jesus. But I was the only one. As I struggled "one day at a time" without using food as a form of substance abuse, there wasn't a Christian in sight.

For a long time, I thought it was because God wanted me to witness to others, but I quickly learned that was not an option. So why was I here? And how was it possible a secular program was working for me?

In the final analysis, I believe God took me to a 12-step program because (1) I was a food addict and I needed it, (2) I was a compulsive eater and I learned spiritual tools to help me stop, and (3) by isolating me from other Christians, I was forced to focus on God alone. Jesus was allowing Himself to be my only God-solution. Let's face it—addicts tend to swap one addiction for another: heroin for alcohol, alcohol for cigarettes, cigarettes for food, food for people. I needed to be saved from replacing food with another powerless but tempting idol. He would not allow me to replace a food addiction with a person, even in the form of friend or sponsor.

My journey to healing would be me and Him. Alone together, fixing my little food problem, because I could no longer do it by myself.

My Little Food Problem

Until this point, I thought of my eating challenges as "my little food problem." This implied it wasn't a big deal, so why would I keep praying about it? God had more important world events on His to-do list than to fuss around with my dinner plans. Besides, food really didn't affect me that much except that I was fat. I can always lose weight, right?

Except I couldn't.

Unhealthy food and food behaviors were a much larger issue in my life than I gave them credit. How did I finally come to this conclusion?

It was much harder to fix than I ever dreamed.

I didn't know how to think about food.
I didn't know how to feel without food.
I didn't know how to pray about food.

I was born knowing how to eat, but I hadn't learned how to eat well. I had no idea how to be faithful with my food so that I could eat and have a strong faith and be full. I needed to master how to eat for wellness and learn how to be food faithful.

There's a video going around on social media where the tune "Can we skip to the good part?" plays, and the medically obese girl raises her palm to cover the lens. When she pulls her hand away, she reveals that she is healthy and fit. Isn't that nice for her?

Not my story.

Time was the mechanism and the fire God used (and still uses) to burn away the garbage in my life.

My food issue was a *spiritual problem* because I was going to food before I was going to God. Using food was how I got through life and "did it myself." I was learning that I didn't function well without fortifying with food first and that was a problem. Giving power to food that I should have only ever given to Jesus was destroying me. I love God, and I have faithfully followed Him since I was five. But when I had any feeling at all, good or bad, I went to food first, then I prayed. This was the root ball of my "little food problem." Not the food itself, but the fact that I allowed my needs first to be met by food and to be met by my Savior second.

"Thou shalt have no other Gods before me." (Exodus 20:3)

Food was an idol. But how was I going to remove an idol that's necessary for life?

The Choice

One day, exhausted from needing food, wanting food, weighing food options, eating, and not eating, I decided to take a nap.

In my dream, I was sitting inside a domed dirt hut by myself in the dark. The walls and floor were mud. I was crouched in a pile of food and covered in the stench of someone who hadn't showered or seen the light of day in decades. I felt flabby, gross, and hated myself, but I was alone with my food, and that was what mattered.

Even if I wanted to leave (which I didn't because the food was here), I couldn't risk anyone seeing or judging me. So, I stayed. Here in this dank place, I could eat all I wanted and be alone. Don't bother me; I'm binging.

Then I jumped at a gentle touch on my arm. I looked up, stunned. Jesus was in my hut! What? Why would He come in here? The place was disgusting.

He helped me off the floor, led me out the door, and we walked into the daylight together. I shielded my eyes from the bright sun. It had been a while.

As my eyes adjusted, Jesus helped me stand tall and cleaned me up and gave me new white clothes. No sign of crackers in my hair, no mud under my fingernails, and no chocolate mustache. I was shiny and smelled great. Arm in arm, He led me away from the hut.

I had a decision to make. Would I go with Jesus or back to my food?

I walked away from the hut with Jesus by my side.

When I awoke, I sat up and realized I had to choose. It was the idol of food or Jesus. I could not have both.

How had I missed this?

The Lord was parenting me one-on-one, telling me He loved me, and He would help me leave my unhealthy food behaviors behind. With this vision in mind, I knew He would help me escape food oppression and strongholds, so I started asking Him for help with every little thing. I asked and asked some more, and He ALWAYS always always always answered me.

"No temptation has overtaken you except what is common to mankind. And God is faithful; He will not let you be tempted beyond what you can bear. But when you are tempted, He will also provide a way out so that you can endure it." (1 Corinthians 10:1)

A Fork in the Road

Over time, God helped me identify my addictive foods: magical foods I believed would "save the day." I noticed I was eating those foods before talking to God and how that choice (to *go to food first for peace and then God*) allowed food to pull me away from my true Savior, Jesus.

Subtle? Yes.
Devastating to my relationship with God? Yes.
Physically and spiritually deadly? Absolutely.

From that point on, I practiced asking Jesus for help first, listening for His answer, and trying it His way first. Jesus would sit on the throne of my life, not hot buttered bread.

I remember one time I was staring at a plate of food. It didn't feel like enough, but it never did. It was, in fact, a healthy dinner portion.

The truth is, no matter how much food I had, I never perceived it as "enough." I felt like I was done eating after the first three bites and started to panic at the thought of an empty plate. I couldn't see the food for what it was; I could only see it for what I needed it to be—a never-ending pile of feel better.

I prayed, "Lord, let it be enough," which had become a regular prayer of mine. I asked "Father, how will I remember that every time I eat, I'm at a fork in the road—choosing life with you or death with food? How will I ever remember the choice I have and to choose you?"

I looked down at the table, and the whisper in my heart that I have come to recognize as the Holy Spirit said, "How about your fork? When you see your fork, remember you're at a fork in the road." I laughed. God has such good ideas.

This is one of the first times I remember God showing up to solve a food problem I had with a practical tool that would help me in any food situation.

"But the Advocate, the Holy Spirit, whom the Father will send in my name, will teach you all things and will remind you of everything I have said to you." (John 14:26)

Another time, I asked the Lord to help jog my brain out of compulsive eating when I opened the refrigerator.

The Holy Spirit brought to my mind a plastic bear about the size of a milk carton gathering dust in our game closet. I thought, "I could put that bear on the top shelf of the fridge to remind me of the Revenant and pray before I eat." The bear had its arms up in an aggressive stance, mouth open in a roar, teeth bared. Perfect. With that, the ferocious bear migrated to a new temporary home on the top shelf of our fridge without so much as a sweater.

Later that day, my husband was rummaging around the kitchen. The refrigerator door opened, and I heard him yell out in surprise. My husband is 6'5". Maybe the bear was scarier at eye level.

"What is this?" He laughed and pulled out the bear.
"It's to remind me to pray before I eat."

"I'll say!" He laughed, and we both had a good chuckle. He still jokes about his reaction and says every person who goes on a food journey with me should get a bear for their fridge.

"We scare because we care." - Monsters Inc.

Throughout my time in the food addiction program, I had sponsors that came and went. Ultimately, however, I considered the Lord my lead sponsor. I made my commitments to Him, my confessions to Him, and my plans for eating and food with Him. People in program were shocked at my "recovery" (read: weight loss.) It was evident from the outside looking in that *something* was working.

What was my secret?

Step one: I came to believe I lost control with food.
Step two: Jesus could and would help me.
Step three: I prayed, listened, and followed Jesus when it came to my food behavior, and He was making me new.

"Therefore, if anyone is in Christ, the new creation has come: The old has gone, the new is here!" *(2 Corinthians 5:17)*

Stronghold Foods

Six months into recovery from food addiction, I woke up and decided I wanted to pick up and eat a flat of cinnamon rolls after I took the kids to school. Before my recovery, I went to the store on the regular and bought a 12" circular pan of frosted cinnamon rolls, ate them all, and destroyed the evidence. I had cleaned up my diet from baked goods in general, but today I was willing to give up the weight I'd lost, the hard work and dedication I'd invested, along with my self-respect, to eat cinnamon rolls with mounds of cream cheese frosting, no fork required.

I was reminded to pray. SIGH.

"Fine, Lord. Fine. I'll pray."

He asked me two questions.

1) What is happening in your life that you would give up everything for cinnamon rolls? I mentally scanned my life's current events. The day before, I received word that my mom was diagnosed with a terminal illness. The Lord reminded me this was not a small problem and to trust Him before cinnamon rolls.

   Good point.

2) Then He asked me, "Would you want the rolls without frosting?"

   Weird question, Lord, but OK, I'll go along. I considered.

   "No, Lord. I would not like to eat the cinnamon rolls without frosting."

I waited for His answer.

"Maybe frosting is a problem food."

NOOOOOOOOOOOO. Lord. NO. NOT FROSTING. UGH. SIGH. NO, NO, NO.

(See me flopping onto my bed, flailing around throwing a sizable tantrum.)

Chips, rice, pasta, ice cream, alcohol, and baked goods were all off the table for the moment, one day at a time. But it didn't dawn on me how attached I was to frosting... until God revealed I was to sacrifice all my progress and confidence to consume its colorful, creamy decadence.

The Lord was on my side. First, He cared for my heart hurt. Then He provided His insight and wisdom. He didn't condemn me but asked intriguing questions that made me think.

The Lord doesn't speak to me in an audible voice as He may for some. For me, the Lord's voice is like a friend talking with me in my heart. I know it is Him because I am not that wise, and I'm not that kind to myself. I beat myself up; He does not condemn me. He is my Father, friend, strength, joy, and salvation.

And thanks to Him, I was now aware frosting had too firm a grip on my heart. I considered my relationship with frosting throughout my life. Frosting is at birthdays and funerals. Frosting is at church and school functions. Frosting is at uncomfortable events and warm gatherings filled with love. My husband hand-fed me frosting at our wedding after smearing a bit on my nose. Turns out, frosting plays a significant role in human relationships. Frosting is a major league life player. Was it even possible to live a full life without frosting?

Yet, the enemy was using frosting to destroy my body, and I never saw it.

"The thief comes only to steal and kill and destroy; I have come that they may have life, and have it to the full." (John 10:10)

"Be alert and of sober mind. Your enemy the devil prowls around like a roaring lion looking for someone to devour." (1 Peter 5:8)

The Lord showed me that if frosting was a tool being used by the enemy to steal my life, destroy my life, and ultimately kill my life ... it had to go.

Breaking Up with Unhealthy Food

What now? I needed a healthy action to replace eating frosting. I prayed and called my sponsor. She told me this story:

To catch monkeys, African trappers are said to cut a coconut in half, clean it out, and put an orange inside. Then they close the coconut and attach it to a tree. Next, they make a hole in the coconut big enough for a monkey's empty hand to pass through but not big enough for the orange to come back out. When the unsuspecting monkey slips a hand into the coconut to grab the orange, he can't escape because he is gripping the orange. The trapper slings a net over the monkey, and he is ensnared. All because he couldn't let go of the food.

Frosting was my orange.

She suggested I write a "break up letter" with frosting and let it go. At first, I thought this was the silliest idea I'd ever heard. But so is eating an entire sheet cake by oneself, so I gave it a shot.

I started by telling frosting what it had meant to me and how it had been a good friend. I wrote about the difficult events it got me through and how much it still means to me when I'm lonely. I thanked frosting for the good times and even for showing up at my wedding and being a special part of cutting the cake with my beloved husband.

Then I told frosting how it was hurting my body and that it was time to break up. I told frosting the relationship was over.

This is the letter I wrote to frosting:

Dear Frosting,

I need to let you go. It's been really fun hanging out in good times and bad over the last 44 years. You are a reliable and sweet friend, and I love you, but you are hurting me. Even the idea that we can't be together makes me sad, depressed, and angry. I want to find some way we can continue. But you take me to a place of dark oblivion. You are pretty, and you come in so many light, playful, and happy colors, and shapes. You always invite me in, and you don't cut me off. You let me be myself and escape with you. You make me feel better, and I light up with happiness and joy—my spirit lifts, and I get a rush every time you are around! You are a reminder of happy times, celebrations, graduations, and new babies. You are there even in the worst of times … like funerals and death. You are available to comfort me at a work party or church party or family party or friend party, or school party when I am extremely uncomfortable and feel lost and confused, and shy.

But I don't need you anymore.

If I am at a party and I feel stressed, I can pray or call a friend. I don't need you to make it easier. If I need to induce happiness, I know how to create joy in other ways. I also know that I need to feel and work through sadness, anger, loneliness, frustration, and other uncomfortable feelings by praying, writing, talking about it, or working out. If I need to celebrate, I have learned other ways like dancing, laughing, picking up some flowers for the house, getting a pedicure, or taking a walk with a friend. If I need to mourn, I now realize you cannot fix grief. I must go to my Jesus and ask Him for help. I can write, I can talk to my husband or a good friend.

I know now that you are exactly as your name says—you are only a frosting. You can cover, but you cannot change or heal. And that's really what I need, to be changed and healed … I WANT to be changed and healed. You work against that in my life. You became too important, and now I have no choice but to let you go and say goodbye. Goodbye.

Julia, 2016

There ended my love affair with frosting.

Writing this letter helped me let go of frosting. Of course, food is an inanimate object, and so from a logical perspective, a letter like this may seem ridiculous. However, there are foods with which we have a special bond, and for me, breaking my bond, or stronghold, with frosting started with this letter.

Next, I talked to God about the letter and asked Him to help me find replacements for frosting. There are not many replacements for frosting itself, but there are healthy non-food replacements to mend the cracks in my life I was filling with frosting. Also, God brought to light information about frosting. One interesting fact He revealed to me through my research was that I was seeking a "sugar shock," which is a sugar high that dramatically improved my mood for a moment, like a hit of cocaine. Yikes. I was taking hits of a drug named frosting.

Turns out, letting go of frosting would improve my overall health as well. Studies show that sugar is killing us slowly by lowering our HDL "good" cholesterol levels, increasing triglyceride levels, and causing diseases like diabetes, obesity, heart disease, and poor oral health and tooth decay, which is now also being linked to poor health in the entire body, not just the mouth.

But my big win? Inviting God to help me overcome my love and need for frosting opened a larger world of real relationship with Him and others, which has increased my self-worth and blessed me with better physical and mental health. I do eat a little bit of frosting now and then. I don't enjoy it like I did; I can leave it on a plate or not eat it at all. It does not have the hold over me that it once did by the grace of God.

It took saying no to frosting for me to realize that only the Lord can do for me what I was expecting from food. As an inanimate object, no amount of food can ever FIX the problem I'm facing. It's just *food*. God is the one with the power to change life, save life, and give life. God alone.

With frosting behind me, I spent 1.5 years in program, lost 60 pounds, and even started sharing at meetings. But there was little tolerance for the name of Jesus, God's only Son and the only Savior.

The foundation of the Big Book is the Bible. Since God's Word is true, it follows that the life lessons taught in the Big Book work whether or not the Bible is credited. However, we don't just need tools for sober living, we need to be saved, and salvation only comes through faith in Jesus Christ. In the recovery rooms of Los Angeles, I could not talk about Jesus unless He was lumped in with all the other idols in the "higher power" line-up, and this was something I could not bear.

Christian Addiction Program, Here I Come!

As I lost weight, people noticed. Hours of fighting food demons went by slowly for me, but to someone I hadn't seen in months, my body transformation happened fast. A lot of Christian friends wanted to know what I was doing, so at one point, I broke down and invited ladies from church to a meeting.

The "gods" named as a higher power that night caught my friends off guard. For example, one person told us how Pat the Panda, his higher power, helped him avoid eating cartons of cannoli left on the kitchen counter after Cinco de Mayo. My friends left the meeting confused, shocked, and disappointed.

I felt bad for going to a "secular" program that made my Christian friends run screaming like Kevin escaping the Wet Bandits. Maybe I *was* in the wrong place after all.

I decided to try out a Christian addiction program at a local church.

The "pride check" learning curve was big for me at this time because some Christians tend to judge, it wasn't anonymous, and the meeting was held at a church where I knew people. Plus, all the vices were lumped into one meeting so when I pulled up and parked next to someone who was going to the sanctuary to decorate the Christmas tree, that person saw me head to the meeting, and didn't know if I was co-dependent, gambled, or boiled crack in a spoon. One time, I was a little late picking up my kids from the childcare, and the volunteer said, "*You people* need to learn how to be on time." Her contempt burned like a hot poker to the heart of this lasagna-loving lady.

Since this church format included all kinds life challenges, I met people recovering from many addictions and hurts … but few if any were there for disordered eating. So, when the heroin addict next to me asked, "What are you in for?" and I said, "Overdosing on pizza," everyone laughed. A funny joke until stacks of gold crusted pepperoni pies show up for the post-meeting social complete with cookies, caffeine, and crème brulee creamer.

I needed a sponsor and asked several women. They all said no. I really wanted this program to work, but it just wasn't clicking for me.

Ultimately, I decided this meeting was not a good fit for me personally because they served food. I could get over being judged by insensitive Christians. I couldn't sit in a vulnerable environment for two hours, listening to all the serious challenges people faced (including my own), then head up to the large group meeting and win against decadent food that would make all the bad feelings go away.

I compare the food served after the meeting to the dead man's heart in Edgar Allen Poe's short story *The Tell-Tale Heart*. The food waiting for me after the meeting, like the dismembered heart buried under the floorboards in the story, seemed to have a heartbeat I could not ignore. It called me, distracted me, and promised to make it all better when this was all over—but it was death. I couldn't concentrate during the recovery meeting when I knew my sinful salve waited at the after-party. It was like closing the meeting in a bar and expecting the alcoholics not to do tequila shots with everyone else. I didn't trust myself, and I knew that it wasn't anyone's problem but mine.

Why do I share this? Not to slight this program at all. This recovery format works miracles for many people. My point is, if you've ever felt like you can't find a safe place either at church or outside of church to get help with your "little food problem," I get it. I was stuck in between only two choices,

1) recover at church with food in my face, or

2) recover with Jesus at a program that didn't want me to say His name.

Not willing to let food defeat me at church, I dragged myself back to the secular rooms of recovery. I reached a healthy weight, had tools to manage my food, and picked up some sponsees. I began speaking and made the best of it. But I knew this wasn't sustainable if I couldn't tell people what Jesus had done for me—and what Jesus alone could do for them if only they would trust Him. There had to be another way.

I was finally healthy, off medication, and succeeding at behavior modification. My kids were thriving. I had cute clothes and felt mentally and spiritually fit. I even started praying about writing a book.

Then everything changed in an instant.

A Slice Down the Middle
January 7, 2018: 46 years old

You know what happened next. I fell to the ground in excruciating pain, was rushed to the hospital and emergency surgery.

The moment where this book began, and my life almost ended.

My husband paced the waiting room for four hours as my surgeon, "Dr. Lifesaver," rinsed two liters of infection out of my gut. There were no holes in my colon, and no organ had burst. He couldn't find anything that would have triggered the event, so he stapled me back together and sent me to the ICU, still in grave danger. The team of doctors were baffled with no explanation for my sickness, and the infection was not resolving. My husband stayed in a chair next to me sleeping, eating, and playing praise music. I was in and out of lucidity. The nurses were kind but concerned. I was not turning a corner.

At one point, an infectious disease doctor marched in, and I heard through a morphine haze that I was not responding to antibiotics, the infection was raging in my body, and I was dying. The only option they had not tried was a form of penicillin. Why? Penicillin makes my throat swell up and sends me into anaphylactic shock. I'd never taken an actual allergy test, but the last time I took penicillin, the doctor threw the bottle in the trash and ordered me NEVER to take it again. Now they were telling me it was my only hope. "The good news is," they hedged, "if your throat closes up, you are in the best possible place to get treatment."

Translation: I would die without it, and I might not die with it.

I'll take "might not die," Alex, for $1000. By the grace of God, my body responded positively, and the infection began to resolve. (I went in for an allergy test months later, hoping to learn that I wasn't allergic to penicillin after all. Turns out … I am allergic.) Praise God for His miracle of protection and healing.

Getting my strength back meant lifting myself out of bed and attempting short walks. My body was weak, and the pain in my midsection was excruciating. They warned me not to rip my sutures, but I had to move—what if I fell or tore something important? My caregivers were also concerned one of my lungs would collapse. The nurses insisted I exhale into a contraption that floated a ping pong ball in the air and gave me a lift goal. Was my ball hiding a 50-pound weight inside? I fought for each centimeter of increase. The pic line in my neck was an infection concern, and my hair smelled awful. A strong, no-nonsense nurse named Luda helped me out of the bed, and we walked the ICU hallways together. We started out with a goal just to make it out my door and back to bed. "Good job!" she encouraged. The next time we'd shuffle one door down. Two doors down, I witnessed a man dying of a collapsed lung while they notified his family. I started making more of an effort with that 50-pound ping pong ball of mine. Soon, I walked all the way to the nurse's station, and they waved as my open-air pajama parade passed by. Luda was relentless and kind, and I learned that getting better was committing to very small steps forward even though I was afraid; it hurt, and sometimes I didn't make it as far as I had before.

You may be in a very difficult situation with your health. Remember, when you are suffering, small steps forward are making a difference. We only heal one step at a time, and those steps can be grueling. The foundation of healing and strength is small, difficult, consistent steps.

When the infection cooled down, I was transferred to a standard hospital room. It was there that one of my best friends came to visit and stood with me as I looked at the wound for the first time. I was bloated and bruised, and the incision was long. Looking at myself stapled and maimed, I started to weep. I am so thankful Lyndy was there with me that day. I couldn't have processed the reality of that heinous, jagged gash alone. My husband was at work, and I could have waited to look at it with him, but I was terrified to witness his reaction at the same time I was experiencing my own. I know he loves me no matter what (and I know that now more than ever). But at that moment, I needed to see it first, and I couldn't do it by myself.

When the surgeon went in to operate on that awful night, he wasted no time saving my life. A clean cut was not his concern. As a result, I was alive, but a jagged reminder ran an inch above my belly button to below my hip. My stomach was severely bloated, crusted with blood, bruised, and oozing.

I was finally happy with my body, and within a year of achieving that long-awaited body confidence, I faced Frankenstein's monster in the mirror that day.

I wept, and my friend didn't say a thing; she stood by me and did not react. She sat with me and hugged me while I cried. She didn't flinch, joke, stare, comment, or try to make light of it. She simply stayed with me while I processed.

What was I going to do? All I knew was I had to get out of the hospital and become strong and healthy again. The doctors said there was only one thing standing in my way.

I had to fart. Someone call the church prayer chain.

It's cute how much control we think we have over our bodies until we need it to do something like toot. I could not flatulate to save my life. Literally.

What's more, I was not allowed food or water until there was proof of poof.

I prayed and walked and prayed some more. I blew into the spirometer and consumed hours upon hours of Property Brothers reruns. Watching Scott and Drew transform fixer-uppers into dream homes distracted me from my sorrow, proved twins can become millionaire besties, and confirmed you can't underestimate the power of a colorful couch pillow to brighten up a rumpus room. Seasons aired, and meals came and went (for my roommate), but my gut was a ghost town.

The "down there" dead silence concerned me deeply. Not just because I wanted to go home, and not just because I wanted to eat. I desperately wanted my colon to be OK.

"Just keep taking steps forward," I'd tell myself. First, I stepped out my door as Luda taught me. Then to the neighbor's door and next around the nurse's station, once, twice, three times, then four. I began to explore other nurses' stations at all hours of the night, soon without a walker. I got to know the staff, and they encouraged me, saying, "You'll be out of here in no time with your determination!" But my abdomen unnerved me with its hollow, dead calm.

Specialists assured me that my colon was healing, resting, and would wake up. Due to the trauma, however, I was concerned it was damaged and would not.

People were praying for me. The nurses were cheering me. But after three days in the ICU and three days in a hospital ward without so much as a flutter of movement, I was frightened, and my heart was desolate.

In the middle of the night on day five, I started to cry. I had not eaten, and my doctor would not allow water. If I begged the nurse, she would sneak me a tiny ice chip or two. Don't tell anyone. My mouth was dry as sand, and there was nothing to be done but wait.

Pushing myself gently to a sideways sitting position in the middle of a graveyard shift, I determined once again to get up and move. Tears dripped down my face. Everything hurt. The night nurses were on lunch, my husband was home sleeping, and I was alone.

"Who will walk with me?" I cried out to the Lord in a silent prayer.

And I saw Him, in my mind's eye, sitting at the end of my bed.

Jesus.

He said, "I'll walk with you."

I got up and walked the halls with Jesus. I smiled a lot on that walk in the middle of the night with Jesus next to me. We enjoyed making the rounds together, and I understood in that moment how much I needed company and comfort. Jesus came and gave me an abundance of both with a bonus of peace.

"Peace I leave with you; my peace I give you. I do not give to you as the world gives. Do not let your hearts be troubled and do not be afraid." (John 14:27)

When I got back to my bed, I did the "sit and scoot" back into a lying upright position … and the ol' tailpipe kicked into gear and backfired.

I have never in my life been so happy for a fart. I cheered, I laughed, and I rang the nurse buzzer like a celebrity judge on America's Got Talent. My colon had been raised from the dead, and there is no doubt it was Jesus who brought it back to life.

Thank you, Lord, for companionship, comfort, and big ol' juicy farts.

Speaking of juice, they brought me all the apple and orange drinks I wanted with a side of soup. I think it was soup.

Praise God from whom all blessings flow.

As Craig and I signed the discharge papers and grabbed my parting gift—the spirometer—Property Brothers chatted in the background. I looked down at my body. Could this broken-down fixer-upper be made into a dream house? I sincerely doubted it. Either way, I had a gut feeling it would take a lot longer than six to eight weeks to find out.

Healing Stage 1

My belly was so disfigured that I rarely looked at it and never took a photo. I wish I had a picture now, but the times were alarming, and I could not bear the sight of my new reality.

The seven-inch vertical slash had staples and two drains. I took meticulous care of the incision; nevertheless, it became infected.

Dr. Lifesaver ordered a home nurse. There was only one home nurse in our area. Tall and greasy, he arrived with dusty medical bags and reeked of cigarette smoke. As someone who has suffered with OCD, you can imagine my horror. I had to lie on my couch while he dressed my wound. I never once looked at the aberration that took center stage on my body. He told me it looked like I had two bullet holes connected by a long gash, and it was infected.

Enter: the wound vac.

A wound vac is a marvelous invention that uses suction to drain the wound so it heals faster. Blood and puss are pulled from the wound through a long, clear plastic tube into a hard carrying case you get to take with you everywhere for four to six weeks. It smells like a salty sewer and is too big to hide. On the bright side, the set comes with a black canvas bag that may or may not have been washed since the last person used it.

The unit was booked on a Wednesday, and I needed the vac, foam, and stylish bag before the end of day Friday when my home nurse went off duty. Everything was to be expedited for arrival two to four days later, but the company promised to have it to me sooner. I scheduled the home nurse for the end of the workday, Friday.

The vac arrived mid-day Thursday.
YES.
The foam and tape arrived end of day Thursday.
Right tape, wrong foam.

Let the freak-out begin. I called the company and told them I needed to have the correct foam the next day. They would do their best, but there was no guarantee. I searched high and low for another source. Nothing. It was Thursday night, and I needed it in less than 24 hours. It wasn't possible, the wound vac representative informed me, but they would send it for arrival on Saturday. My nurse was off duty on Saturday. It had to come Friday.

I prayed and prayed and prayed and prayed and prayed and stressed and prayed some more. I needed this foam, and the error was going to affect my health dramatically. I was in a lot of pain; my wound was not healing well, and my fever was going up. Infection was increasing by the hour. This had to be managed yesterday.

I didn't cancel the appointment with the nurse scheduled for late Friday and prayed some more. I called my doctor and the nurse, and my husband. There was nothing anyone could do. I was at the mercy of a shipping company with an impossible deadline.

On Friday, the hours ticked by 11 a.m., 12 a.m., 1 p.m., 2 p.m., 3 p.m.—There was no chance it was coming today. But I prayed for foam.

The nurse was scheduled to come at 5 p.m. It took him about 45 minutes to get to my house, so I needed to tell him by 4:00 if the foam didn't come … 4 p.m. … 4:15 p.m. I didn't call him. I prayed and prayed and paced and prayed and paced. I'd call him at 4:30.

At 4:25 p.m., the doorbell rang.

The mail carrier, the foam, and my nurse (finishing a phone call and stomping out his cigarette) were all out front.

I learned two important lessons from this experience.

1) If the Lord can arrange a mailed package to arrive just in time against impossible odds, He can literally do anything.

2) My home nurse was not the person I would have chosen in a lineup. However, he gave me excellent care and was calm and respectful in every way. If I called him freaking out about sudden pain or problems with the vac, he always picked up, even when he was eating dinner with his kids, and helped me with gentle wisdom.

"Man looks at the outward appearance, but the Lord looks at the heart." (1 Samuel 16:7 NASB)

The Lord knew who He had planned in advance to care for me, including an educated and experienced nurse, starting over in a new country with his family. A man addicted to cigarettes and helping people. I judged him with my standards, not God's. I'd work on that because I knew that there would be a long line of medical professionals in my future, each hand-picked by God for His purpose in my life. Ultimately, I would trust the Lord to heal me and protect me, not people.

What does this have to do with my food journey? I'm glad you asked …

Due to being on an IV for almost a week, all meds, stress, and food not tasting right yet, I was skinny. In fact, I could finally cross one leg over the other, make a leg pretzel and flap my flats.

One of my friends told me I was too thin. Yes! I had fantasized about someone telling me that my whole life.

We have a digital frame in our living room that flips through years of family photos. When a picture of me in the first few months after emergency surgery would pop up in the frame, do you know what I thought to myself?

"I'm so glad I lived." Nope.

"That was a cute shirt." Nope

"I need to get down to THAT weight again." Yep.

Fun fact, my lowest weight after the hospitalization and initial recovery wasn't even close to my "goal weight." After being septic, almost dying, chopped stem to stern, living in the ICU and the hospital on an IV for almost a week with no food, and then not eating much for weeks because food tasted bad … I *still* never got to my "goal weight."

But I looked gaunt, and that was good enough for me.

Healing Stage 2

About six months into my recovery, I could lift, turn, and even get in some mild exercise. The bloating had receded, but the infection left the scar wide, long, and keloid. My abdomen was numb now that the pain had ceased, and I was constantly flinching and guarding it, careful not to do any damage that might tear or change the healing trajectory.

Then one day, my stomach popped out. Suddenly I looked like I was in the 4th trimester of pregnancy. What had I done??

Dr. Lifesaver diagnosed a hernia. My abs had split in two and needed to be repaired. As soon as my insides "cooled down" in another three months, they could go in and fix it.

Lucky me, I got to enjoy looking pregnant without being pregnant for three months until my body was ready for another invasive surgery.

True to his word, nine months after the first surgery, Dr. Lifesaver put my abs back together again. I got new drains and all. Oh, joy.

Three months later, I felt another "pop" in my upper ab that I recognized as another hernia.

I went to three doctors and had a CAT scan. They all assured me there was no hernia.

But it was there. I felt it.

When running Save the Ta-tas®, I would often encourage women to "be their own advocate" because I learned from survivor stories that medical professionals helping us simply can't experience what is happening in our bodies. They are knowledgeable, but they don't live in our skin. If they won't listen, we need to tell them *again*.

Furthermore, on the day my gut exploded, no one believed it wasn't the flu until I was almost dead. Fact is: sometimes medical professionals get it wrong.

Now was the time to learn from my experience and advocate for my own health. If my doctors in network were not going to find the problem, I would have to pay for the doctor who would. I had experienced a hernia pop; I knew what it felt like, and I was sure it had happened again.

After months of research, I found a surgeon who was able to locate the hernia and repair it. I went right into physical rehab mode, again. Soon after, my hair started falling out in clumps. The hits kept coming. My dermatologist told me hair loss was a common reaction to anesthesia, and it would grow back.

One setback after another came and went as I settled into the long haul of creating a balanced recovery and a strong and healthy body. I invested in a trainer who specialized in elderly people recovering from surgery. She was merciless when I complained.

"Edith crushes 20 curtsy lunges and never whines like you. Edith is 92."

Well, if Edith can do it.

One Fear Remained

No one ever discovered why the infection happened in the first place, and I was concerned that my gut would explode again. Countless follow-up visits with various specialists assured me I was fine.

But was I?

Reading my Bible one morning, a verse jumped off the page and hit me so hard in my soul I actually flinched.

"Is anyone among you in trouble? Let them pray. Is anyone happy? Let them sing songs of praise. ***Is anyone among you sick? Let them call the elders of the church to pray over them and anoint them with oil in the name of the Lord.*** *And the prayer offered in faith will make the sick person well; the Lord will raise them up. If they have sinned, they will be forgiven. Therefore, confess your sins to each other and pray for each other so that you may be healed. The prayer of a righteous person is powerful and effective." (James 5:13–26 NIV)*

The Lord told me to follow the instructions laid out in this verse.

"No, Lord." I said, "I'm not doing that." The thought of asking the pastor and the elders of my church to help me was too embarrassing. "They don't have time for me! Besides, all the doctors said I was fine."

I wouldn't do this. It was my imagination that God was suggesting it, and I put it out of my head.

But the Holy Spirit kept reminding me in the gentle, loving, and consistent way He does.

"James 5. Ask them."

One Sunday between services, while I was working at the bookstore, one of the elders of the church walked by. The Holy Spirit reminded me to ask him if the elders at our church prayed for people James 5 style.

"Still not comfortable with that," I told God, shaking my head.

But I knew I had to approach the elder.

"Fine." I negotiated, "If he walks by again AND makes eye contact with me, and smiles, then I'll ask."

Five minutes later, he walked by, made eye contact, and smiled.

"Fine." I grumbled.

Waving him down, I asked, "Do the elders pray over people here, like James 5 style?"

"We do!" he said. "We do it really early in the morning, and sometimes it takes a while; be prepared to wait."

I sent an email that afternoon and the pastor invited me to the next meeting in only a few days' time at 6 a.m.

That was fast.

My husband had an early call into work and could not come. I REALLY wanted him with me, but I had to take the opportunity offered. We decided it was okay for me to go by myself, and the morning came, I got up early and prepared to leave. Trembling nerves made it hard to breathe.

Craig was getting ready by the mirror and got a text. His call time had been pushed. He could go. HE COULD GO!! This was amazing news and an exhilarating answer to my silent prayers. My breathing normalized a bit, and we headed over. The living room was filled with godly men and our lead pastor. I only knew two of them.

After I sat down, God told me to tell them about my OCD and my compulsive overeating.

"NO, LORD! I'm here for prayer for my gut and my medical issue. Not that! Oh, please, Lord," I begged. "Don't make me tell them about that."

"Ask them."

No, no, no, no, no, no. Now I was sweating and shifting in my chair. My husband asked me if I was alright.

Not really.

Our lead pastor, Michael, introduced us and explained why we had joined the meeting. He told the story of my undiagnosed infection and asked if the elders would follow James 5 and pray for me.

"Let's pray," he said.

TELL THEM.

"Wait ..." I whispered. "There's one more thing ... since we're here."

"Sure," Michael nodded.

"I also have OCD and I am a compulsive overeater. Would you pray for that too? Since we're here ... praying ... anyway?"

I fought back my tears of shame.

Michael smiled warmly, putting me at ease. "Hmm." he said, "Maybe that's why you're *really* here. Let's pray."

One of the elders anointed me with oil, and Michael instructed the elders to pray silently for me and ask the Lord what He might reveal while worship music played. After silent prayer, they would lay hands on me and pray for me out loud and share what the Lord showed to them, if anything. I sat in the circle and waited. We followed the instructions found in James 5:13-26. After a song and silent prayer, laying hands on me and my husband, the elders prayed and prophesied over me. I was concerned about what they would say, what the Lord would tell them. But the words blessed me with unspeakable joy. They prayed for healing, they prayed for me to know God loved me, and they prayed for perseverance and faith. They saw pictures of the Lord holding me. They prayed for healing for my body, my OCD, my compulsive eating, and blessing for my future. They were kind, compassionate, loving, and honest. It was a landmark moment in my life that I will always remember with a thrill, gratitude, and joy.

This was the moment the Lord had for me when He asked me to be obedient to James 5. Exhilarated, we thanked the elders and left.

He Gives Sight to the Blind

As I went through my day, I noticed my eyes were different. To be more specific, I saw food differently—physically and spiritually. Had I experienced healing?

The best way I can describe the change is this: Before God healed me, I saw piles of food as small and "not enough." I could perceive an entire table of food as "not enough." I couldn't take one bite from a full plate without immediately fearing it was already gone. No matter how much food it was, *it wasn't enough*. This is how I physically "saw" food with my actual eyesight. It was as if my whole life I had thick plastic faux lenses covering my eyeballs, distorting how I saw food.

After God healed me, I could see a plate of food at face value. A single portion. Enough for two. Satisfying or fluff. Also notable, for the first time, I saw food as too sweet, too rich, necessary, or unnecessary. Never in my life had I *ever* considered food too sweet, too much, too rich, or *unnecessary*. My view of volume changed; I valued quality over quantity. I started sharing food (true story). Until this day, I was unaware that I had a warped visual perception of food. Now, I was experiencing a tangible vision change linked to spiritual restoration that allowed me to see food realistically.

I didn't tell anyone for a couple of weeks what I was experiencing because I didn't fully understand how the healing was unfolding. It multiplied like wildflowers popping up in a grassy meadow as I experienced different eating situations, but I didn't yet understand the extent of the change. Had scales really fallen off my eyes? I hadn't been blind, and there were no physical scales to show anyone. But the truth remained when it came to food. I had been blind, and now I could see.

Back to School
October 2018

"What next, Lord?" I asked.

"Don't neglect the gift." That sounded like a familiar Bible verse, so I looked it up.

"Do not neglect your gift that was given to you through prophecy when the body of elders laid their hands on you." (1 Timothy 4:14 NIV)

I would (1) endeavor to manage my eating habits, likes, and dislikes in a healthy way and (2) find an avenue to help others break free from the bondage of food as well. Let the adventure begin.

My friend Monica met me for lunch at the local coffee shop to catch up. She's a therapist, so I spilled my heart out to her about how I wanted to share my experience overcoming food addiction to help others do the same, but I had no credentials.

"Why don't you become a Health Coach?" Monica asked.
"Health Coach? What's that?"

She explained that Health Coaching is like a certified, professional health cheerleader. That sounds like my cup of cappuccino!

I began training to become a Certified Functional Medicine Health Coach and graduated in August of 2019. Over the next five months, I studied fervently and sat for the National Board Exam in early February, 2020, and within a few weeks, Covid hit our country. I was in the last group to sit for the exam until after the Covid lockdowns ended, and I had passed.

When the world came to a screeching halt, I continued my education and earned additional certification in the areas of mental health and emotional eating, as well as weight loss.

I took on clients and began coaching any chance I could get. It absolutely amazed me how God's Word and our health collide for maximum life and joy. I loved sharing my newfound knowledge with anyone who would listen.

Get Up and Go Time

Between 2020 and 2022, Covid regulations made life unpredictable. Maybe the kids were at school, maybe they were home on Zoom trying to go to school. Maybe Craig was at work, or maybe he was home tinkering. The world turned upside down, rattled about, and when it flipped again, there was a lot of clean-up and catch-up. Amidst it all, the Lord asked me to get up early and write.

Mornings aren't my favorite, but He helped me. I made coffee and sat in front of my computer sometimes as early as 4:30 a.m. I asked Him to be present and give me ideas and clarity. Day after day, I would crawl out of bed at o'dark thirty and brew a cup with one eye shut. The Lord was faithful, and this program is a result of His plan for the material as I clacked away on the keyboard.

When I finally thought I had enough words for a book, I printed it, separated it into major themes, and noticed I had twenty chapters—two Bible studies, each 10 weeks. I went to work with rewrites and shared a chapter with some close friends who know the Bible and love the Lord. After getting their comments, I set out to finalize the first draft of the program.

As a wife and mom dedicated to my husband and kids, it has taken time to get everything on paper. In fact, when I was planning to finish this draft yesterday, my daughter broke a bracket on her braces. I hit save, and as we ran out the door, I told my husband, "If this story ever gets told, it will be a miracle."

If you're reading this: Look! A miracle.

Who I Was *Is Not* Who I Am
2022: 50 years old

My life is God's handiwork in progress.

"Therefore, if anyone is in Christ, the new creation has come: The old has gone, the new is here!" *(2 Corinthians 5:17)*

I couldn't stop eating.
Now I can.

Food controlled my life.
Now it doesn't.

I didn't want to participate in life without food.
Now I am excited about many activities that have absolutely nothing to do with food.

Food was destroying my body.

Now I intentionally use food to promote good health.

I used to body shame myself.
Now I believe that God handcrafted me for a good purpose.

I couldn't process emotion without food.
Now I can endure all things with God by my side, and food isn't even a factor.

The scale used to guide my life.
Now the Lord guides my life, and I do not allow the scale to dictate my day or my value.

Food was my #1 source of happiness.
Now I experience an abundant life because Jesus, not food, is my source of overflowing joy.

I couldn't stick to any diet program.
Now I succeed at my health goals without diet programs.

I could never maintain weight-loss victories.
I have maintained a healthy weight since 2016, all glory to God.

Food was used as a tool by the enemy to control me.
Now food is a tool I use to bring glory to God in my life and body.

Today, food is a gift, *not a god*.

And my goal weight?

My goal weight isn't my goal any longer. Why? Because now, my purpose is to have a relationship with God, not the scale. The scale is not a higher power guiding my life and choices and self-worth. It is only a box on my bathroom floor showing a number that is one piece of data about a complicated body doing many different things, some I can control and some I can't.

The scale will never say, "WOW, Julia, you're perfect today!" But when I stand before God, He tells me I'm dearly loved, intentionally created, and He has a purpose for my life.

He says the same to you.

"For we are God's handiwork, created in Christ Jesus to do good works, which God prepared in advance for us to do." (Ephesians 2:10)

Are you ready to stop being controlled by food and be liberated from food obsessions and unhealthy food behaviors? Would you like to have a deeper relationship with God than you ever dreamed possible? He loves you and has the power to set you free.

Transformation *is* possible. He is doing the impossible for me, and He can do the impossible for you.

"Now to him who is able to do immeasurably more than all we ask or imagine, according to his power that is at work within us, to him be glory in the church and in Christ Jesus throughout all generations, for ever and ever! Amen." (Ephesians 3:20–21)

Are you ready to start an amazing adventure to overcome your food strongholds for lasting health and joy? Awesome. It's time to break free from food chains for good.

Let's do this.

Song of preparation: "What You're Worth," Mandisa & Britt Nicole

Dear Food,
I love you.
I hate you.
Don't leave me!

Workbook 1

"The Lord is gracious and compassionate,
slow to anger and rich in love."
Psalm 145:8

Chapter 1

Is This really Going to Work?

What we'll talk about:

Acknowledge skeptical feelings when starting a new food management plan.

Why it matters:

God cares about our relationship with food and His involvement changes everything.

Wisdom from the Word:

"Forgetting what is behind and straining toward what is ahead, I press on toward the goal to win the prize for which God has called me heavenward in Christ Jesus."

Philippians 3:13-14

Recommended Song of Preparation:

"No Impossible with You" by I Am They

Welcome!

Thank you for picking up this Bible study and getting started. Judging by the fact that you're here, I'm going to hazard a guess you've been down this road before. What road? The leafy green vegetable-lined path to weight loss Shangri-La. And it's been torture.

The last thing you want to do right now is go on a diet … again. It might be more fun to poke your eye out with a mascara brush. Now that I mentioned it, if you're really honest, you doubt it will work anyway. Why? You've tried and failed so many times you know it's going to take a miracle to shed the weight you want gone. Besides, you're not really sure God's in the "weight-loss business."

You have a point.

If it were as simple as "calories in, calories out," you'd already be jammed into those goal pants strutting around the supermarket instead of glaring at their dusty, dark home in the corner of your closet. Stop taunting us, skinny jeans, we're coming for ya!

Let's do this differently.

Let's celebrate more often.
Let's encourage each other.
Let's invite God into our journey.
And let's make a new way in the wilderness (and by "wilderness," I mean "the pantry").

Here's the good news—this isn't a "diet book." I'm not going to tell you what to eat, when to eat, or how to eat (insert sigh of relief here). What we will do is discover how to succeed with eating goals, whatever that may look like.

Now that that's out of the way, let's talk about what you'd like to get out of this experience.

What's Your Dream?

Take a moment to draw a picture of **Future You**. This will show the victorious you once you've achieved your health goals. This is a picture of you after winning the battle. It's OK if you can't draw; you'll understand what you meant, and the "you" in the picture will feel so good, they won't care either! Once you draw a picture of yourself, draw circles in the empty space around your body. We're going to call these "benefit bubbles." Inside the bubbles, write all the benefits you are living out and experiencing because of what you've accomplished. Here's an example of what your final picture might look like:

Future Me

Here's an example from my life:

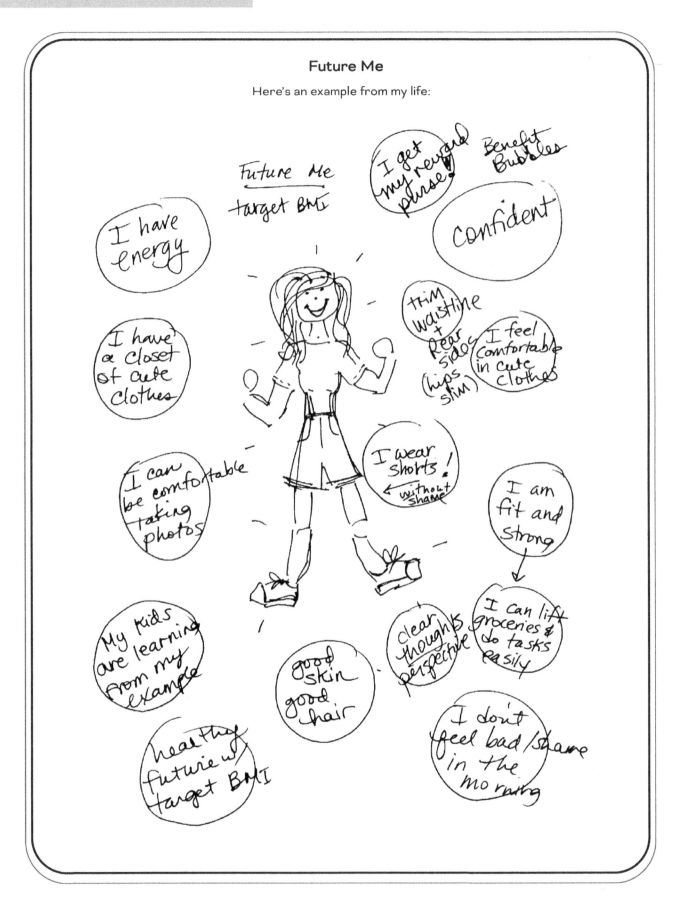

Future Me:

Now it's your turn.

Draw a picture of "Future You," the person you envision being once you have reached your goals. Around the picture, draw all the benefits you are experiencing; these are your "benefit bubbles." Put this picture in a frame or tape on a mirror so that you can regularly see your future vision.

Define Your Personal Success

What a fantastic vision you have for yourself! Well done.

Examine your "**Future Me**" drawing.

1. What powerful motivator stands out as a reason you desire to lose weight and/or pursue healthier food habits? _____

Maybe you have more than one important reason. Great! Here's more space.

_____   _____
_____   _____

It's critical to define our own success when it comes to our health journey. Why? Because it's very difficult to reach a winner's circle we haven't defined. In a horse race, the Winner's Circle is an enclosed, defined area where the jockey and the horse go after the race to receive their reward. If there was no finish line for the horse and jockey, why would they participate? How would they know they won? If there were no Winner's Circle, what would motivate them to run with tenacity, power, and commitment? Just like a horse and jockey, we need to map out our very own Winner's Circle. We need a vision. We need a finish line. We need a reward. We do this by defining our personal success.

Often, we believe the finish line, success, and our reward are the same and/or come at the same time. In day-to-day life, the reality is they may be simultaneous, or they may occur along the way as separate, celebratory milestones worthy of celebration.

2. How do you define the following for yourself in the area of food and health?

I would consider _____ my finish line.
I would consider _____ success.
I would consider _____ my reward.

3. Explain when you expect these to occur. At the end? Together? Separately? Write down some of your expectations.

_____
_____
_____
_____
_____

4. Who has defined your finish line? You? A parent? A program? The Lord? Pray and write down thoughts as you consider defining your finish line.

_____
_____
_____
_____
_____

We Know What We Want to Do. Why Don't We Do It?

Great job defining your future self, success, and what victory looks like for you. Winning looks so good, so why is it so hard to attain?

If you're like me, you know exactly **why you want to stop** unhealthy eating. The real challenge is you don't know **why you can't stop** unhealthy eating. Oh, the exasperating enticement that is food!

Are you ready for some good news?

You're not alone. There are a lot of us who struggle with eating challenges. As foodies, we can all relate to how painful and shame-inducing this vice can be. Take comfort; the struggle is common and human.

In Romans 7:15–25, Paul (a very committed and godly man in the Bible) says,

"I don't really understand myself, for I want to do what is right, but I don't do it. Instead, I do what I hate … I have discovered this principle of life—that when I want to do what is right, I inevitably do what is wrong. I love God's law with all my heart. But there is another power within me that is at war with my mind. This power makes me a slave to the sin that is still within me. Oh, what a miserable person I am! Who will free me from this life that is dominated by sin and death? Thank God! The answer is in Jesus Christ our Lord." (New Living Translation)

5. How can you relate to Paul when it comes to your food challenges?

_____
_____
_____
_____
_____
_____
_____
_____
_____
_____
_____
_____
_____
_____
_____
_____
_____
_____
_____
_____
_____
_____
_____
_____
_____

There Is a Path to Victory

We are all tempted, and, at times, we all succumb to temptation. Isn't it a relief to know that we are not alone? We all fail. We all need help, and I would take it a step further and say that we all need *supernatural* help. For those of us who know the Lord, the fantastic, lifesaving news is—**we have a solution**. Specifically, our Father in Heaven has a solution. Help is just a prayer away. Let's ask Him to help us because He will help. Every time. How do I know? He promises in His Word that He will.

1 Corinthians 10:13 says:

> "No temptation has overtaken you except what is common to mankind.
> And God is faithful; He will not let you be tempted beyond what
> you can bear. But when you are tempted, He will also provide a way
> out so that you can endure it." (New International Version)

I remember looking at my dinner plate with healthy portions on it when I first started my weight-loss journey with the Lord. I stared at it and wept because I didn't believe it was going to be enough food. It looked so small. I had some health issues associated with extra weight, and I knew I was at critical crossroads. I was either going to eat for life or eat food that was destroying me. Through tears, I asked the Lord how I was going to remember that every time I sat down to eat I was facing a fork in the road. He brought my eyes to my fork and gently suggested to me that my fork could remind me I was at a fork in the road. "Great idea, Lord!" I thought. Ever since then, my fork has been a reminder not only that I'm at a fork in the road when I eat but also that the Lord is with me every step of the path to victory.

6. Have you ever prayed for a "way out" or asked God to help you escape a food temptation? Explain.

_____
_____
_____
_____
_____
_____
_____

7. How might you apply 1 Corinthians 10:13 to reach your vision for successful, healthy eating?

_____
_____
_____
_____
_____
_____
_____
_____
_____

Describe a food-related temptation pitfall.

8. My temptation pitfall:

_____
_____
_____
_____
_____
_____

9. Write a prayer asking God for a way to escape this pitfall. If God gives you an idea, write that down as well.

_____
_____
_____
_____
_____
_____
_____
_____

10. When you consider starting this food journey to overcome the power that food and unhealthy eating has over your life, what could be different this time around? Ponder this in light of 1 Corinthians 15:57:

"But thanks be to God, who gives us the victory through our Lord Jesus Christ."

_____
_____
_____
_____
_____
_____
_____

Chapter 1 Wrap-Up

11. Write down questions you have for God about food, overeating, and your life. Ask Him for insight and wisdom. If nothing comes yet, that's ok. Simply jot down your thoughts as you are praying.

_____
_____
_____
_____
_____
_____
_____

12. What is one thing you can do to apply what you learned in this chapter starting today?

_____

_____

_____

_____

_____

_____

_____

_____

You're on your way. It's time to run a new race, right into your very own winner's circle with the Lord by your side.

Promise Prompt:

Cut this verse out and post it in a place you visit often to remind you that God is helping you overcome unhealthy eating.

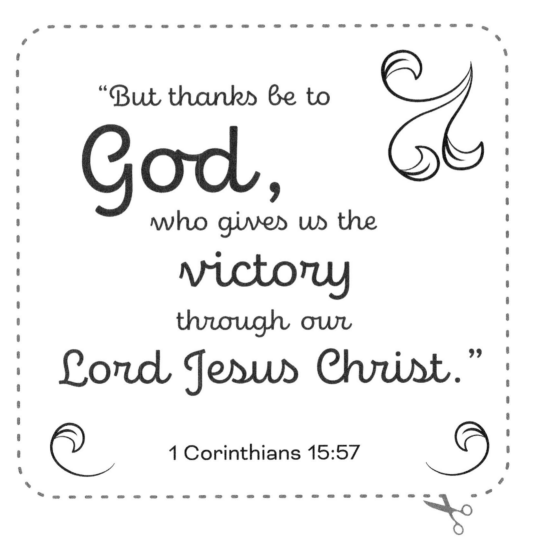

"But thanks be to **God,** who gives us the *victory* through our *Lord Jesus Christ.*"

1 Corinthians 15:57

Journal Your Thoughts

Here is more space to write.

Date: ....

....
....
....
....
....
....
....
....

I am thankful for: ....
....
....

Chapter 2

To All The Nachos I've Loved Before

What we'll talk about:

Our history with food.

Why it matters:

Identifying harmful eating behavior that is guided by family history, past hurts, and life events helps us rewrite the story.

Wisdom from the Word:

"And I am sure of this, that He who began a good work in you will bring it to completion at the day of Jesus Christ."

Philippians 1:6

Recommended Song of Preparation:

"Fires" by Jordan St. Cyr

Share a success story about applying Chapter 1 to your life.

_____
_____
_____
_____

Well done!

Our Cheetos-Checkered Past

Those of us who love eating often have a complicated history with food. Whether food has been our best friend or worst enemy, fond memory or painful regret, we just can't get enough. The good news is our past doesn't define our future because God has promised to complete the *good work* He is doing in us.

If we're going to step into that plan, we need to acknowledge the importance we have given food in our lives. Once we have a clear vision of the hold food has on our hearts, we can better adjust where necessary.

For example, food in my life has played the role of what I would describe as an abusive boyfriend. Were I to write the tale of our juicy and dangerous affair, it might go something like this:

"When we started out, food rocked my world. Every experience was amazing. Then, food started to hurt me. So, I cut it off cold turkey. But it called to me at all hours, and I just couldn't stay away. We reunited in a whirlwind. Midnight rendezvous, weekend getaways. Bliss. Then it hurt me again. I took some time off, but I got lonely. Sigh. I let food in again. It was slow at first, and I was cautious. But food quickly took over my life as it always does. The truth is, I don't want to be physically and emotionally harmed because of my relationship with food anymore, but I feel trapped and don't know how to escape."

Your "relationship" with food might look like mine, or it may be different. Food for you might fit the description of a caring mother, a loan shark, a judgmental best friend, or a part-time lover.

1. Imagine food is a person in your life. Describe what kind of "person" food might be and the nature of your relationship. For example: *"Food is like a caring mother. It nurtures but also smothers me."*

_____
_____
_____
_____
_____
_____
_____
_____
_____
_____
_____

If you're like me, you're asking yourself, "How did I get involved with food like this again?" and, more importantly, "How do I break free?"

We can discover useful answers to these questions by examining our food history.

Below, you'll see a worksheet titled: **My Food History Timeline.** Fill out the timeline and consider your relationship with food over the years. How has food affected your life, health, and well-being? Let's explore when your love for food started, how it grew, the weight you've lost and gained, as well as the victories and challenges you have had right up to where you are now. Next, we're going to use our timeline discoveries to help us create a healthier future.

Let's pray:

Dear Lord, please be with me as I fill out this timeline. Please encourage me and provide insight and wisdom as I seek to understand better my relationship with food, how it affects my life, and how it affects my relationship with You. Thank you for being by my side and helping me recover from unhealthy eating.

<blockquote>
"For the LORD gives wisdom; from His mouth come knowledge and understanding."
Proverbs 2:6
</blockquote>

Add anything else you'd like to say to the Lord before getting started.
_____
_____
_____
_____

Wonderful. Now, let's fill out your **Food History Timeline**.

My Food History Timeline

Use this space to write down any family history of obesity, weight-related or nutrition-related health issues:

....
....
....
....
....
....

Use this space to write down any family history of addiction:

....
....
....
....
....
....

Use this space to write about signs, symptoms or diseases you may be experiencing: (ex: high cholesterol)

....
....
....
....
....
....

On the timeline below record your food history. Include events like the first time you gained weight, or went on a diet, when you have gone on diets, weight losses and gains, and major life events such as college, marriage, divorce, abuse, illness diagnosis, surgeries, childbirth, accidents or grief .

Birth

My Food History Timeline

Use this space to write about people, or other factors (past or present) that have impacted your eating practices: (ex: I had to finish everything on my plate, medication)

....
....
....
....
....
....
....
....
....
....
....
....
....
....
....
....
....

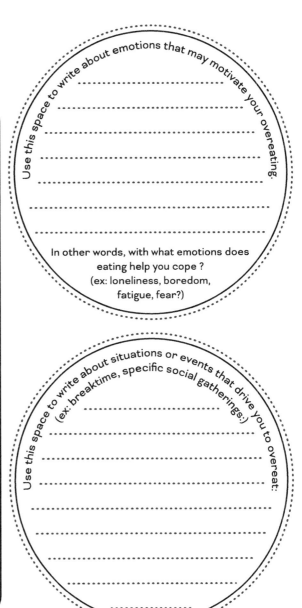

Use this space to write about emotions that may motivate your overeating.

In other words, with what emotions does eating help you cope ?
(ex: loneliness, boredom, fatigue, fear?)

Use this space to write about situations or events that drive you to overeat:
(ex: breaktime, specific social gatherings:)

Present Day

67

This isn't an easy exercise and you finished it. Way to go!

2. What trends do you notice in your **Food History Timeline**?

_____
_____
_____
_____

Identifying when you have been vulnerable in the past allows you to prepare in advance for success the next time you are vulnerable in this way.

3. Pick a trend from your **Food History Timeline**, maybe it is a repeat event such as "when I am lonely, I gain weight." Write down the trend and one idea to stay on your health plan next time it surfaces.

Trend: *(Ex: I get lonely and I eat ice cream out of the container.)*

_____
_____

My idea to help me stay on my health plan next time the trend surfaces*: (Ex: Next time I feel lonely I will call Kathy and go out to coffee with her. I will also call Gina and ask her to go on a walk with me instead of eating ice cream.)*

_____
_____

Look at you rewriting your food story! Good job. Let's rewrite some more.

Intentionally Creating a New Path

We're born, and we eat. This gives us a false sense that eating is automatic, second nature, and we should know how to do it. Functionally, that is true. We innately know how to eat. What most people don't consider is that we all have to *learn* how to *eat well.* Healthy eating is a life skill that takes personal assessment, data collection, research, practice, and trial and error ... and what we eat may need to change based on life stages, body changes, and current health conditions.

4. Examine your food timeline. What old rules, practices, and habits are you following without questioning?

_____
_____
_____
_____

5. Which of these old rules, practices, and habits are no longer useful?

_____
_____
_____
_____
_____

6. Which old rules, practices, and habits are harmful to your health and well-being?

_____
_____
_____
_____

7. What new and healthy eating practices could you switch out for former unhealthy old rules, practices, and habits?

For example:
I could change the rule "clean your plate" to "I choose to eat a healthy portion for my body."
I could change "eating in secret" to "portioning out the food and eating it out in the open."

Now it's your turn:

I could change: _____ to _____.
I could change: _____ to _____.
I could change: _____ to _____.

8. Is there an event in your past that re-circulates in your thoughts and triggers unhealthy eating? Describe the event. Then write about the power this event still holds over you.

Event:

_____
_____
_____

Power the event has over me (and my eating specifically):

_____
_____
_____

9. How might processing this discovery with a trusted friend or counselor help you better succeed in your health journey?

_____
_____
_____

Rewriting the Story

"And I am sure of this, that He who began a good work in you will bring it to completion at the day of Jesus Christ." Philippians 1:6 (English Standard Version)

10. How does this verse resonate with you after filling out your **Food History Timeline**?

_____
_____
_____
_____

11. How might you and the Lord begin to rewrite your food story to create a healthy food future?

_____
_____
_____
_____

12. List weight loss and food management successes you wrote on your timeline that (1) worked and (2) you'd enjoy trying again.

_____
_____
_____
_____

13. Write down *new* things you'd like to try to rewrite your story and create a healthy food future.

_____
_____
_____
_____

14. Go back to your **Food History Timeline** and highlight all the times God did something amazing. Share one of the memories here:

_____
_____

If you get sad, feel regret, pain, or other uncomfortable feelings swell when you remember the timeline this week, consider what the Lord has brought you through. He is the hero of the story, not food. He was your hero then, and He will be your hero again.

> "See I am doing a new thing! Now it springs up, do you not perceive it? I am making a way in the wilderness and streams in the wasteland." Isaiah 43:19

Chapter 2 Wrap-Up

Well done with the **Food History Timeline**. Keep it handy because we'll refer to it again. Next time you want to eat in a way that isn't in line with your health "success" from Chapter 1, consider this timeline. Ask yourself what healthy action you could take instead to rewrite your food story.

15. What is one thing you can do to apply what you learned in this chapter starting today?

_____
_____
_____
_____

Promise Prompt:

Cut this verse out and post it in a place you visit often to remind you that God is helping you overcome unhealthy eating.

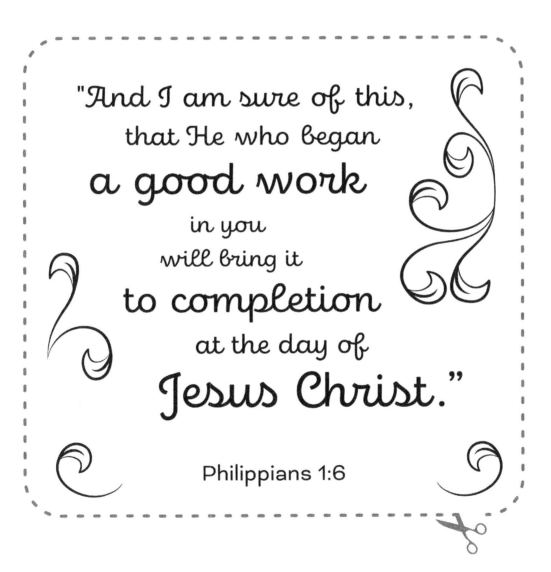

"And I am sure of this, that He who began **a good work** in you will bring it **to completion** at the day of *Jesus Christ.*"

Philippians 1:6

Journal Your Thoughts

Here is more space to write.

Date: ....

....
....
....
....
....
....
....
....

I am thankful for: ....
....
....

Chapter 3

Why Can't I Find "Thigh Gap" In My Bible Concordance?

What we'll talk about:

Discovering God's vision for our health.

Why it matters:

God's plan for our bodies comes with a lifetime soul-satisfying guarantee.

Wisdom from the Word:

"For you have been bought for a price: therefore, glorify God in your body."

1 Corinthians 6:20

Recommended Song of Preparation:

"Every Step of the Way" by Cade Thompson

Share a success story about applying Chapter 2 to your life.

_____
_____
_____
_____
_____

Well done!

Finding a Lost Treasure

When I was 16, my mom gave me her diamond cross necklace. It's tiny and delicate, and to this day, I've not seen one like it anywhere. I've worn it most of my life for the past forty years.

One day, I went to check the clasp and move it to the back of my neck, and I noticed the necklace was gone! It had fallen off. I was heartbroken, and I looked everywhere for it for days. It didn't turn up. I prayed and prayed but did not find it. Later that week, as I was walking into the house after the day the gardeners mowed the front lawn, I noticed something glinting in the sun. It could have been water, but it didn't rain that day, and the sprinklers had gone off hours earlier. As I reached down into the grass, I saw it was the necklace! I was overjoyed to have found my lost treasure. I even got a new chain for it, and I wear it to this day.

1. Tell a story about a treasure you lost and then found.

_____
_____
_____
_____
_____

You Are Jesus' Treasure

Jesus loves you deeply. He created you; He knows you, and He is fully aware of what your body can and can't be according to His great love and plan for your life. Your body, whether sick, healthy, wrinkled, or missing a few parts, is of the utmost importance to the Father.

He picked you. He wants you, and He's got a job for you. He purchased you with a very high price (the life of Jesus) to bring you out of the land of darkness and into His kingdom. He came after you, like a shepherd finding a lost sheep, you are His treasure, and He rejoices over your presence in His family! You are His. Even if you lose your way with food, He will come find you.

Read Luke 15.

2. What do these parables tell you about how important you are to the Lord?

_____
_____
_____
_____
_____

Flip back in your "**Future Me**" drawing.

3.   Write down desires you have for your health, well-being and future.

_____   _____
_____   _____
_____   _____
_____   _____

Great! Your desires are important to the Lord.

In fact, heart desires are directly linked to the Lord.

Psalm 37:4 states:

> "Delight yourself in the Lord and He will give you the desires of your heart."

4.   What does it mean to "delight in the Lord"?

_____
_____
_____
_____

5.   How do *you* "delight in the Lord"?

_____
_____
_____
_____

If the desire of our heart is to be healthy, it follows that delighting in the Lord is a crucial step to reaching our health goals.

My "Why," or God's "Why?"

We often search and search for *our* "why" (our core reason for sticking to a healthy living plan) without ever asking the Lord to reveal His "why" for our body health and wellness. We don't ask Him what health goals He might suggest. We don't ask Him why He thinks those goals are important – or if He has a different health goal for us than we have for ourselves. We forget that He loves us, wants to help – and is our best ally for success! As God's kids, doesn't it seem reasonable that our "why" would naturally include learning about and following God's "why" for investing in our body and our health?

One way to "delight in the Lord" is to trust Him enough to invite Him into our thoughts, desires, and ideas, co-creating with Him our future plans (and goals) for health and wellness.

6.   Have you ever asked God what *He* wants your body to be? Explain.

_____
_____
_____
_____
_____
_____

7. Not sure how to start talking to God about your health and wellness path? Here are some ideas to get the ball rolling:

   a. Ask God to reveal His plan for your body. "Dear Lord, please show me in a way that I can hear and understand what your will is for my body, my self-image, and my body confidence."

   b. Read and meditate on Psalm 139:14. Ask the Lord to speak to you about how it applies to your personal body and health situation.

   "I praise you because I am fearfully and wonderfully made, your works are wonderful,
   I know that full well." Psalm 139:14

   c. Write a gratitude list about the body God gave you. What has it done for you? What has it survived? What has it adapted to and allowed you to do? What is special about it? Spend time thanking God for the body He gave you and attached your spirit to. Ask Him to reveal more about how this relates to your current situation and what you can do to help advance His plan through your life, your spirit, and your body.

8. After completing one or more of these exercises, jot down some of your thoughts about what you think God is telling you about what *He* wants your body to be and how He thinks you should view your body.

_____
_____
_____
_____
_____

Sorting Through a World of Expectations

What are some expectations the world puts on you that define your value and, as a result, disrupt your confidence? For example, the customs of this world might tell us we need to have pillow-soft lips, perfect skin, and extra points for a thigh gap.

9. Write down the "world's" expectation, and circle Y if you agree with it or N if you don't. If you're stuck in the middle, write your feelings on the lines below. Sometimes we know something isn't true, but we *feel* like it is.

Ex: The world says I shouldn't have flappy underarm skin. I agree Y / N / Maybe

_____I agree Y / N / *Maybe*
_____I agree Y / N / *Maybe*
_____I agree Y / N / *Maybe*
_____I agree Y / N / *Maybe*

When the world's values come in conflict with ours or our own thoughts and feelings get confused, or we find ourselves agreeing with questionable values, it's good to have the Bible as a solid reference for truth, meaning, and purpose.

Romans 12: 2 says:

> "Don't copy the behavior and customs of this world, but let God transform you into a new person by changing the way you think. Then you will learn to know God's will for you, which is good and pleasing and perfect."

Let's apply this verse to our health goals and body image.

What would change if we transformed …

What I think my body should be ——> *enjoying the body God made for me*
What the world says I should be ——> *valuing what God made me to be*

Let's change the way we think by clicking off the world's input on how we should perceive our body and our value. Click. You got that influence turned off? Good. Now, let's turn on our willingness to see and believe God's good, pleasing, and perfect will for our health, body, and worth.

We'll start down this path with prayer, then read His Word and ask for counsel from the Holy Spirit.

Let's pray.

Dear Lord,
Thank you for helping me with my health and wellness journey. I ask you to transform me into a new person by changing the way I think that I may learn your good, pleasing, and perfect will for my life and body. I know you made me, and you love me. Help me to have confidence in YOU, even when I don't have confidence in myself. Please give me discernment, strength, and joy as I live my life all to your glory. Amen.

10. Write down any thoughts you have after praying this prayer.

_____
_____
_____
_____
_____
_____
_____
_____
_____
_____

God and Body Image

Our Father is incredibly creative. Variations in design and what some consider "defects" may not be insufficiencies or negatives to God at all. In fact, flaws imbue interest and authenticity.

11. List physical flaws you feel you have that negatively affect your life.

_____   _____
_____   _____

Read the following verses.

Read Genesis 1:27:

> "God created mankind in his own image, in the image of God He created them; male and female He created them."

Read Psalm 139:13–16:

> "For you created my inmost being; you knit me together in my mother's womb. I praise you because I am fearfully and wonderfully made; your works are wonderful; I know that full well."

12. What do these verses tell you about how you were created?

_____

_____

_____

_____

_____

_____

13. What do these verses tell you about your value as God's intentional creation?

_____

_____

_____

_____

_____

_____

Consider resentments you may have toward God regarding your body.

14 Write some of these disgruntled feelings below.

Dear God, sometimes I don't understand why you made me like this:

_____

_____

_____

_____

_____

_____

Read the following verses:

Ephesians 2:10

> "For we are God's handiwork, created in Christ Jesus to do good works, which God prepared in advance for us to do."

Ecclesiastes 7:13-14

"Consider the work of God, for who can straighten out what He has made crooked?"

Romans 9:18–21

"But you are a mere human being. So who are you to talk back to God? Scripture says, 'Can what is made say to the one who made it, 'Why did you make me like this?' Isn't the potter free to make different kinds of pots out of the same lump of clay?'" (New International Reader's Version)

2 Corinthians 12:9

"But He said to me, 'My grace is sufficient for you, for My power is made perfect in weakness.' Therefore, I will boast all the more gladly about my weaknesses, so that Christ's power may rest on me."

15 How much say and control do you have over your body? Think in terms of what it does and what it is, and what it can't and can be. Explain.

I have control over:

_____
_____
_____

I don't have control over:

_____
_____
_____

16. What do these verses tell you about any mistakes or errors you think God might have made when making you?

_____
_____
_____
_____
_____

Rick Warren once said, "God won't give us anything that isn't useful." In light of the scripture you just read, consider the following:

17. Why are your weaknesses important?

_____
_____
_____
_____
_____

You were intentionally made by God. Let that settle into your bones for a minute. Everything about you was made on purpose by Him. You are a work of art.

18. What does Ephesians 2:10 tell you about why God made you the way He did, even if you're not so sure you like it?

_____
_____
_____
_____
_____

Refer back to personal body characteristics you consider flaws.

19. How has God used something you consider flawed to help you do good works He planned in advance for you to do?

For example, "I don't like my belly, but God used it to bring my child into the world."

_____
_____
_____
_____
_____

He's not done yet. There's more life ahead. He's going to continue to use you, as you are, and all the beautiful body parts and pieces you love (and hate) for His good purpose as you partner with Him and live for Him.

20. How does knowing this give you strength to keep fighting and overcome?

_____
_____
_____
_____
_____

21. How can a deeper understanding of your body and God's will for you help you encourage others who struggle with physical and body issues?

_____
_____
_____
_____

Aging with Purpose

Aging is hard. You can't roll past 40 without a few bald spots, scrapes, and/or bladder control issues. Read the following verses and consider what the Bible has to say about the problems associated with aging:

2 Corinthians 4:16

> "For this reason, we never become discouraged. Even though our physical being is gradually decaying, yet our spiritual being is being renewed day by day. " (GNT)

1 Samuel 16:7

> "The LORD does not look at the things people look at. People look at the outward appearance, but the LORD looks at the heart."

22. How can you look at aging differently through the lens of God's Word?

_____
_____
_____
_____
_____
_____
_____

The Body Gift

Let's examine how the Bible teaches us to value, view, care for and use our bodies.

1 Corinthians 6:19–20

> "Or do you not know that your body is a temple of the Holy Spirit within you, whom you have from God? You are not your own, for you were bought with a price. So glorify God in your body."

Ephesians 2:10

> "For we are God's handiwork, created in Christ Jesus to do good works, which God prepared in advance for us to do."

Colossians 3:17

> "And whatever you do, whether in word or deed, do it all in the name of the Lord Jesus, giving thanks to God the Father through Him."

1 Corinthians 10:31

> "So, whether you eat or drink or whatever you do, do it all for the glory of God."

1 Corinthians 9:26–27

> "So, I run straight to the goal with purpose in every step. I fight to win. I'm not just shadowboxing or playing around. Like an athlete I punish my body, treating it roughly, training it to do what it should, not what it wants to. Otherwise, I fear that after enlisting others for the race, I myself might be declared unfit and ordered to stand aside." (Living Bible)

23 What does scripture tell you about your ultimate worth, regardless of anything else you might think or believe about your value (yesterday, today, or tomorrow ... unconditionally)?

_____
_____
_____
_____
_____

24. What is the ultimate purpose of your body?

_____
_____
_____
_____
_____

25. What is the purpose of what you do in life, including eating and drinking?

_____
_____
_____
_____
_____
_____

26. How might this purpose be helped or hindered by eating unhealthy food?

_____
_____
_____
_____
_____

27. What do these verses teach about how important it is to God that we take care of our bodies?

_____
_____
_____
_____
_____

28. What level of commitment does God expect from us when it comes to training our bodies?

_____
_____
_____
_____
_____
_____

Read Hebrews 12:11:

> "No discipline seems pleasant at the time, but painful. Later on, however, it produces a harvest of righteousness and peace for those who have been trained by it."

29. What is the cost of disciplining our bodies? What are the rewards?

Cost:

_____

Rewards:

_____

Nice work!

Asking God for a Game Plan

Now that we have a grasp on what God's Word says about caring for our bodies, we're ready to ask the Lord for guidance.

Dear Lord,
As I read Your Word, I have learned a lot about how You made my body, value my body, and want to use my body. (Jot down anything that comes to mind.)

_____
_____
_____
_____
_____

Now, I'd like to ask You, through the counsel of the Holy Spirit and in the name of Jesus, to speak to me and let me know what Your health goals are for me. I ask You to be gentle with me and clear. Help me to understand what You have to say and help me follow You.

30 Use this space to write down what comes to mind in terms of what the Lord may be sharing with you about His health and body goals for you.

_____
_____
_____
_____
_____
_____
_____
_____
_____

Thank you, Lord.
Amen.

Chapter 3 Wrap-Up

God's health goals for you may stay the same and/or change with the seasons according to His purpose. What matters is that you continue to delight in the Lord and invite Him into your heart to share life. Just watch and see how much He loves you as His plans unfold.

31   What is one thing you can do to apply what you learned in this chapter starting today?

_____
_____
_____
_____
_____
_____
_____
_____
_____
_____

Promise Prompt:

Cut this verse out and post it in a place you visit often to remind you that God is helping you overcome unhealthy eating.

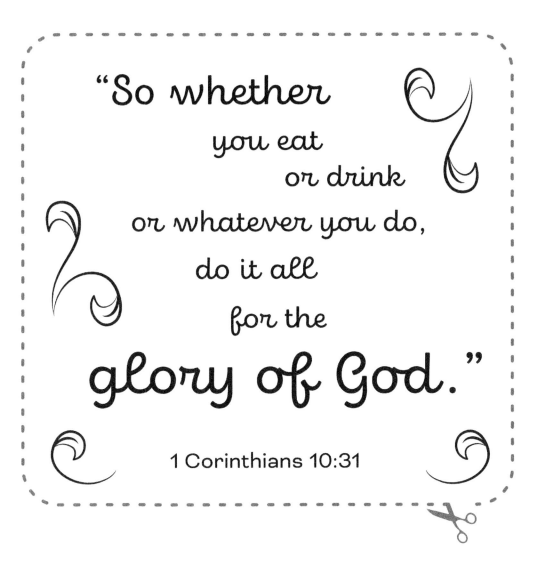

"So whether
you eat
or drink
or whatever you do,
do it all
for the
glory of God."

1 Corinthians 10:31

Journal Your Thoughts

Here is more space to write.

Date: ....

....
....
....
....
....
....
....
....
....

I am thankful for: ....
....
....

Chapter 4

Jesus is the Answer
(What was the question?)

What we'll talk about:

If Jesus really cares and if He's really going to help.

Why it matters:

When we are sure Jesus really cares and really helps, we actually go to Him for care and help.

Wisdom from the Word:

"Come to me, all who weary and burdened, and I will give you rest." -Jesus

Matthew 11:28 BSB

Recommended Song of Preparation:

"My Jesus" by Anne Wilson

Share a success story about applying Chapter 3 to your life.

_____
_____
_____
_____
_____
_____
_____

Well done!

Sunday School Jesus

Growing up as a Christian, I've been to a lot of Sunday School classes. As a middle schooler, we'd slouch in our metal folding chairs, whisper during class, and find it hilarious to answer "Jesus" every time the teacher threw out a question. I am sure the teacher found this just as amusing as we did.

Okay, maybe not.

Sunday School teacher: "Who made the world?"
Smarty-pants middle schooler: "Jesus."

Sunday School teacher: "Who died on the cross?"
Know-it-all middle schooler: "Jesus."

Sunday School teacher: "Who wants you to have an abundant life?"
Punk middle schooler: "Jesus."

Sunday School teacher: "How do you live that life?"
Rowdy middle schooler: "Jesus."

Sunday School teacher: "Who wants fruit punch and a cookie?"
Silly middle schooler: "Jesus."

You see where I'm going with this? (If you answered "Jesus," you would be correct).

As kids, we called this the "Jesus answer" because it was a super simple way to get the question right without thinking or paying attention. Technically, you didn't even have to be listening, especially if you were flirting with the boy in front of you. Not that I know from experience or anything.

The "Jesus answer" worked, but it didn't acknowledge the reason for, the purpose of, or the complexity of the question.

Flash-forward to adulthood … our questions are much more serious. Does the "Jesus answer" still work?

Painful Cries with Unknown "Whys"

When we enter the wild world on our own, and *we're* the adult (when did that happen, where did that huge pile of laundry come from?) the questions of life can be much more complex and painful than most of us would ever have expected.

How do I save my marriage?
How do I raise balanced, healthy children when I'm so flawed?
Why is my parent dying from Alzheimer's?
How do I stop eating so much unhealthy food when I am completely stressed at work?
How can I lose weight when my body chemistry is working against me?
Why did I get the fat genes and the fat jeans?

1. What big question do you contemplate in the context of food and eating?

_____

_____

Food, Pain and the "Jesus Answer"

When it comes to my food issues, I've been given the "Jesus answer" by countless well-meaning Christian friends.

A man named Job in the Bible faced intense hardships. If you haven't read the Book of Job, I highly recommend it. In the depth of his despair, three friends came to "help." They did some things right, like showing up, and at the same time, managed mistakes in judgment that made Job feel worse. Sometimes my friends have been a lot like Job's—hurting me with all the best intentions.

Tell me if you can relate.

Me: "I really struggle with my weight. I just can't seem to lose it and keep it off."

Christian friend 1: "Have you read what the Bible says about gluttony?"

Christian friend 2: "Are you praying about it?"

Christian friend 3: "You just need to want *Jesus* more than food."

Christian friend 4: "Have you 'given it over' to Jesus?"

I've been praying *to Jesus* about my weight and my "little food problem" for almost a half a century. So yeah, I've "given it over" to Jesus, sought wisdom in the Bible, and memorized verses. This kind of advice from well-meaning friends made me want to scream into my pillow or throw my face in a cheesecake, whichever came first.

2. What discouraging word of encouragement can you remember a Christian friend giving you about dieting and weight loss?

_____

_____ (Take a moment to forgive them if you haven't already.)

We have faith, and we believe … so why do these "Jesus answers" leave us ashamed and confused? I love Jesus. Of course, Jesus is the answer to any problem I have, not just food but everything. I know this. *I believe this.*

Nevertheless, I translated the many "Jesus answers" given to me over the years by genuine Christians to mean "If you loved Jesus enough, you wouldn't be fat," or worse, "If Jesus loved you enough, Julia, you wouldn't be fat." As a result, I went to a dark place that left me feeling ashamed, unworthy, and more hopeless than ever. All of which drove me to take more solace in food with each passing day.

I cried into my cheesecake with the question, "If 'Jesus' is the answer, why isn't anything changing?" Then one day, it dawned on me: I knew the answer, but I hadn't asked the Lord to answer my really scary questions.

Really Scary Question 1: *"Will* You Help Me, Jesus?"

Jesus loves us deeply. A youth leader once told me that if I was the only person on the planet, Jesus would have gone to the cross to die *just* for me. That's always been hard for me to imagine, but the Parable of the Lost Sheep seems to support the theory. Jesus' death and resurrection are personal. The cross was for you and for me, and it was a tremendous act of dedicated and sincere love. Do you think He's going to let a "little food" get in the way of His love for you? Not a chance. He's way bigger than this food problem, and if it's standing in the way of us experiencing His love and care, He will show up and help us be "more than conquerors" in Him.

> "In all these things we overwhelmingly conquer through Him who loved us."
> Romans 8:37 (New American Standard Version)

The Answer is YES. Jesus does want to help me, and He wants to help you, too.

For me, coming to believe this with certainty (moving out of head knowledge and into experiential knowledge) meant going to Him repeatedly, asking for help, and seeing what happened. He did show up, every single time, over and over again, saving me. This is what it took for me to finally understand that Jesus was all in.

He does love me, and I am worth His time—as are you. Tears well up in my eyes even as I write this now. How can it be that Jesus could care for me so? But He does, and the same goes for you. You are loved and cherished by God. He loves you, and He will come to your rescue. Confirm it by calling on Him, asking for help, and experiencing what happens next. We must give Him the opportunity to love us by inviting Him into our food problems with faith through prayer. If you're asking if your food challenge is worth His time and effort … *the answer is YES*. The cross showed it, the Bible confirms it, and His work in our lives each day, each hour, each minute proves it.

Jesus cares about your body. Why? Because your body is the temple of the Holy Spirit. *Your body is how He houses your precious soul to do works He planned in advance for you to do.*

Ephesians 2:10 says:

> "For we are God's handiwork, created in Christ Jesus to do good works, which God prepared in advance for us to do."

If your body is being harmed by unhealthy food, of course, He will help you with that challenge. If your unhealthy eating habits are causing you shame or depression, of course, He will help you with that. God made your body. He made it for you, and you are a treasure to Him. Your body matters to God because YOU matter to God.

Read the following verses in light of the question, "*WILL Jesus help me?*":

Isaiah 41:13

> "For I, the LORD your God, will hold your right hand, saying to you, 'Fear not, I will help you.'"

Jeremiah 29:12–13

> "Then you will call on me and come and pray to me, and I will listen to you. You will seek me and find me when you seek me with all your heart."

Hebrews 4:15–16

> "For we do not have a High Priest who cannot sympathize with our weaknesses, but was in all points tempted as we are, yet without sin. Let us therefore come boldly to the throne of grace, that we may obtain mercy and find grace to help in time of need."

Our hope in Him will not disappoint.

Romans 5:5

> "… and hope does not disappoint, because the love of God has been poured out within our hearts through the Holy Spirit who was given to us."

3. How do these verses help you answer the question "*Will* Jesus help me" with my food struggles?

   _____
   _____
   _____
   _____

4. How do these verses ignite hope that things can, and will, improve when you invite Jesus to help?

   _____
   _____
   _____
   _____

Really Scary Question 2: "*When* will Jesus help me?"

Whew! Good news ... Jesus *will* help us. Now we need to know *when* He will help us. Within the hour? Tomorrow? Next Tuesday at 10:03 a.m.? What if a more pressing issue comes up, will He leave and come back later? Will He totally desert me because I ate dessert?

Does Jesus care enough to show up for me when I call on Him in my moment of need, *even* if it's just about a brownie bite?

Consider how the following verses address the question, *"WHEN* will Jesus help me?":

Psalm 46:1

> "God is our refuge and strength, always ready to help in times of trouble."

Psalm 72:12

> "For He will deliver the needy when he cries, the poor also, and him who has no helper."
> (King James Version)

Isaiah 41:10

> "Fear not, for I am with you; be not dismayed, for I am your God. I will strengthen you,
> yes, I will help you, I will uphold you with My righteous right hand."

Psalm 107:9

> "For He satisfies the longing soul, and the hungry soul He fills with good things." (New
> King James Version)

5. What do these verses tell you about *when* Jesus will help you (yes, even with your food struggles) when you call on Him?

_____

_____

_____

_____

_____

6. How do these verses ignite hope that things can, and will, improve when you ask Jesus to help?

_____

_____

_____

_____

_____

Jesus may not take the trouble away; however, there is a powerful purpose in His decision to walk with us through trouble. He is teaching us that by partnering with Him and abiding in His strength, we can endure. This builds confidence in Him, confidence in ourselves, and confidence to handle the future because we know and have seen what leaning on Him can do. His power and trustworthiness change us at a core level and make our light brighter and our much… muchier (to quote *Alice in Wonderland*). We are warriors being trained by Jesus to overcome this dark world with His power. Life here on earth isn't going to stop coming at us, and Jesus is right here, helping us survive and thrive. Without overcoming, there would be no sweet victory. Victory that empowers and refreshes and fills the very fibers of our being with exuberance and joy is vital to our human experience. This special brand of joyous triumph only blooms after conquering something devastatingly difficult in a way that was only possible with the help of Jesus.

Which brings us to the next big question.

Really Scary Question 3: "*How* will Jesus help me?"

Jesus will help us and come quickly to our aid. Yet, there was one more lingering question: *how* is Jesus going to help? In other words, *if I can't see a way out of this, what can Jesus possibly do?*

Let's find our answer in scripture. Read the following verses in light of the question, *"**HOW** will Jesus help me?"*:

Isaiah 40:29–31

> "He gives power to the weak, and to those who have no might, He increases strength."
> (Amplified Bible)

2 Corinthians 12:9–11

> "But He said to me, 'My grace is sufficient for you, for my power is made perfect in weakness.' Therefore, I will boast all the more gladly about my weaknesses, so that Christ's power may rest on me. That is why, for Christ's sake, I delight in weaknesses, in insults, in hardships, in persecutions, in difficulties. For when I am weak, then I am strong."

1 Corinthians 10:13

> "No temptation has overtaken you except what is common to mankind. And God is faithful; He will not let you be tempted beyond what you can bear. But when you are tempted, He will also provide a way out so that you can endure it."

Romans 8:28

> "And we know that in all things God works for the good of those who love him, who have been called according to his purpose."

7. Explain what these verses tell you about *how* Jesus will help with your food struggle.

_____
_____
_____
_____
_____
_____
_____
_____

8. Write down what you need Jesus to help you with regarding your eating journey. Be specific (i.e., not eating after 8:00 at night, hitting the pause button on pudding pops).

_____
_____
_____
_____
_____
_____
_____
_____

9. How do these verses ignite your sense of hope that with Jesus, things can, and will, change for the better?

_____
_____
_____
_____
_____
_____
_____
_____

10. Pray about additional needs you have considering your new understanding that Jesus (1) wants to help you, (2) will come to your aid quickly (is already with you,) and (3) has a solution you might not have considered. Write down what comes to mind as you spend time talking to the Lord.

_____
_____
_____
_____
_____
_____
_____
_____

Resting in Jesus

Coming to the life-altering understanding that we are not alone, not for one moment, because we have a Savior that saves us not just for eternity but for today changes our ability to cope. Once we experience the fact that Jesus can help us, wants to help us, has the power to help us, and is available right now to walk with us through anything we face, we can finally taste peace. As we learn to ask for, seek, and acknowledge His presence, we come to know He is our hiding place, strength, and solution because of His great love for us *personally*. Food as a solution pales pitifully in comparison to the great love and power of our Lord Jesus Christ.

In Matthew 11:28, Jesus said, "Come to *me*, all who are weary and burdened, and *I* will give you rest."

11. Write about how resting in Jesus' great love for you and His presence in your life might give you peace and perspective so that you don't have to go to food for solace.

_____
_____
_____
_____
_____
_____

Food For Thought

Jesus taught us to pray The Lord's Prayer.

Luke 11:1–4

> "Our Father, who art in heaven, hallowed be Thy Name; Thy kingdom come; Thy will be done on earth as it is in heaven. Give us this day our daily bread; and forgive us our trespasses as we forgive those who trespass against us; and lead us not into temptation but deliver us from evil."

Jesus also told us that He is the bread of life.

John 6:35

> "Then Jesus declared, 'I am the bread of life. Whoever comes to me will never go hungry.'"

12. Take a moment as we close this chapter to ask the Lord about the "bread" we need to ask for each day. Just food? The Bread of Life? Write down thoughts that come to mind as you consider what bread you need each day and how to ask for it.

_____
_____
_____
_____
_____
_____

Chapter 4 Wrap-Up

13. What is one thing you can do to apply what you learned in this chapter starting today?

_____

_____

_____

_____

_____

_____

_____

_____

Promise Prompt:

Cut this verse out and post it in a place you visit often to remind you that God is helping you overcome unhealthy eating.

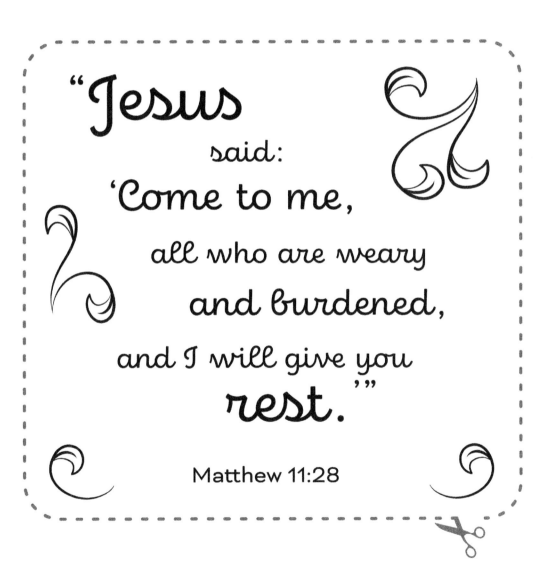

"Jesus said: 'Come to me, all who are weary and burdened, and I will give you rest.'"

Matthew 11:28

Journal Your Thoughts

Here is more space to write.

Date: ....

I am thankful for: ....

Victorious You!

Let's stop right here.
On this page in this book.
To see what you've done,
It's amazing, JUST LOOK!

Your journey's not over,
to conquer the food.
But take heart and be glad
that's no reason to brood.

If we wait to celebrate
or say, "Good job, Me!"
It could be a while,
until Heaven we see.

So right here and right now,
We're going to cheer
Let this victory moment
make you smile ear to ear.

Write your wins down
Big and small too,
It's time to acknowledge
and celebrate YOU!

'Cause victories don't just come
at the end.
Sometimes it's a victory
just to begin.

Successes arrive
at all times, and between
Every victory
each one
Deserves to be seen.

- Julia Fikse

Take a "Victory Lap!"

Celebrate success big or small!

Victory Lap: Pause to celebrate your win. Thank the Lord and tell yourself you did a good thing.
Smile and approve of the progress you are making. Enjoy how good it feels. Well done. You did it!!

Date: ....

Victory: ....

How I feel about myself: ....

Why I did it:
....
....
....

Things that helped me succeed:
....
....
....

How God helped me:
....
....

I have new hope that: ....
....

I could try this strategy again for another win:
....

What I have learned from the victory:
....
....

I am thankful for: ....
....
....

Use this Victory Journal page to start recording your victories!
Download more pages here: www.onesteptowellness.com

Chapter 5

Why Am I So Mean To Me?

What we'll talk about:

Negative self-talk.

Why it matters:

Our minds and hearts can deceive us about us. We need to go to the Word for the truth.

Wisdom from the Word:

"Therefore, do not throw away your confidence which has a great reward."

Hebrews 10:34

Recommended Song of Preparation:

"No Hold On Me" by Matty Mullins

Share a success story about applying Chapter 4 to your life.

_____

_____

_____

_____

What Did I Just Say to Myself?

I remember when I was around 220 pounds and considered going back to the gym. "But," I thought, "I'll be the only fat person there, and everyone will stare and be grossed out by me." Of course, I didn't go. My mean voice in my head kept me from taking an important step forward, and I listened to that inner self-shaming for far too long. When I finally went to the gym, I realized no one cared what I looked like or how I performed except my trainer and me … both of whom wanted me to succeed.

Do you have a big meanie voice in your head like I do?

Here are some things I tell myself:
"Ugh, I'm so fat."
"Why am I so stupid?!"
"I'm a horrible person."
"I'm gross."
"You always fail."

Here are some things my clients tell themselves:
"It's not going to work anyway."
"You're too old."
"Why bother?"
"Does God really care?"
"You're disgusting."
"I'm weak."

We would never utter a word like this to a friend, so why do we say it to ourselves? Welcome to "negative self-talk," sometimes called "the gremlin," and other times "the inner critic."

Negative self-talk has a lot of names, but call it what *we* may, *it* calls *us* "stupid," "old," "worthless," and on occasion, "cottage cheese thighs." I'm not talking about hearing voices, but instead, I'm referring to the inner dialogue that influences our behavior and causes shame and self-sabotage if not remedied. Luckily, we can learn to identify and silence it. Let's shut it down 'cause this gremlin has got to go pronto.

In my life and in the lives of my clients, negative self-talk can pop up in second person (e.g., *"you're* such a dork") or in first person (*"I'm* such a dork"). For the sake of this discussion, I'll call negative self-talk that enters our thoughts via second person *The Accuser*. I'll name the negative self-talk that comes at us in the first person *The Robber*. Let's separate the two and take a closer look.

The Accuser

The inner Accuser's words come at us hard and fast, like a direct hit of an arrow, sinking straight into a psychological soft spot. The way it pops into our heads and how it phrases criticisms is usually a quick, succinct accusation in second person. For example: "You're so stupid."

We may have heard the "You are …" accusations from another human, and it stuck like dirty gum on the shoes of our lives. Or these accusations may have a spiritual source. Either way, there's a very real possibility we didn't think up the original accusation all on our own.

Human Accusations that Wound

"You are …" accusations we recirculate in our minds and hearts may have originated from a person of significant influence in our lives. For example, maybe your grandma once told you, "You're the ugly grandchild." It might have been something a mom said, or a friend, a dad, sister, or aunt. Maybe the sticky condemnation came from someone you didn't know, like a rude boy at summer camp shouting, "YOU HAVE PIG LEGS!" running past, never to be seen again. (This is an actual event from my life, and as a result, I rarely showed my legs until my forties.)

1. Write down "You are ____(accusation)____" phrases that still haunt you, which you can attach to a specific person in your life. They may have said it directly, or it may have been implied.

Accusation: Person who said it:

_____   _____
_____   _____
_____   _____
_____   _____
_____   _____

These are difficult things to remember, acknowledge, and write down. Well done.

Silencing the Accuser Through Forgiveness

Romans 3:23 says, "All have sinned and fall short of the glory of God." Sadly, there is collateral damage with sin. Their sin hurt someone else, in this case, you. Thankfully the damage isn't final, and there is an antidote—forgiveness. Forgiveness robs these accusations of their power because forgiveness replaces their cruelty with grace. Wouldn't you rather have God's grace cover and fill your mind and heart instead of an ugly accusation? Forgiving the people on the "person who said it" list is an important first step to removing their accusations from your inner dialogue.

The definition of forgiveness that works best for me is *"surrendering my right to retaliate or punish the person who wronged me."* This means I hand over "getting even" to God. In my experience, practicing the act of forgiveness is a recurring effort until it's not. I experience forgiveness in a similar way as I experience grief. The feelings of hurt go out and come in like waves of pain. When they are out to sea, I am confident the forgiveness is complete, but they inevitably "roll in" to my thoughts again. When the wave of hurt hits me, I pray for help and intentionally forgive *again*. After repeating this many times, the waves become smaller, and eventually, the day comes when they stop coming back. Forgiveness is a repeated act of obedience, one thought at a time, as the memory or thought occurs. Consider the following verses:

Romans 12:18–19

> "If it is possible, as far as it depends on you, live at peace with everyone. Do not take revenge, my dear friends, but leave room for God's wrath, for it is written: 'It is mine to avenge; I will repay,' says the Lord."

1 Peter 3:9

> "Not returning evil for evil or insult for insult but giving a blessing instead; for you were called for the very purpose that you might inherit a blessing."

Ephesians 4:23

> "Be kind and compassionate to one another, forgiving each other, just as in Christ God forgave you."

Consider how to use forgiveness as an antidote to inner dialogue you rehearse that came from someone else:

2. What good reason do you have, based on scripture, to forgive those who left you with accusatory negative self-talk?

    _____

    _____

    _____

    _____

3. Write down one step you can take to start forgiving someone who has contributed to your inner accusations. (Take a moment to pray for willingness and ideas.)

    _____

    _____

    _____

    _____

4. Pray a special blessing over the life of each accuser you have listed. This is hard, but the promise, according to 1 Peter 3:9, is a blessing from God for you. Write your prayer below.

    _____

    _____

    _____

Accusations from the Adversary

According to scripture, there is another source of condemnation that originates from the dark side of the spiritual realm.

Revelation 12:10

> "And I heard a loud voice in heaven, saying, 'Now the salvation and the power and the kingdom of our God and the authority of his Christ have come, for the accuser of our brothers has been thrown down, who accuses them day and night before our God.'"

1 Peter 5:7

> "Be sober-minded; be watchful. Your adversary the devil prowls around like a roaring lion, seeking someone to devour."

Ephesians 6:12

> "For our struggle is not against flesh and blood, but against the rulers, against the authorities, against the powers of this dark world and against the spiritual forces of evil in the heavenly realms."

In John 8:44, Jesus describes the devil:

> "He was a murderer from the beginning and does not stand in the truth because there is no truth in him. Whenever he speaks a lie, he speaks from his own *nature*, for he is a liar and the father of lies."

Romans 16:20

> "The God of peace will soon crush Satan under your feet.
> The grace of our Lord Jesus Christ be with you."

5. Write down accusing thoughts, "You are ____(accusation)____", that run through your head that you can't attribute to a specific person. Is it possible these accusations came from a spiritual force of evil who is a "liar and accuser" as defined in scripture?

Accusing thoughts:

_____

_____

_____

_____

6. Look at your list above. Is there an accusation written that you know is a lie?Explain.

_____

_____

_____

_____

These phrases aren't your identity. They likely didn't come from you and may not be true or could be twisted truth. Once you have clarity, the Bible teaches us how to fight the lies.

Read Ephesians 6:11–18

> "Put on all of God's armor so that you will be able to stand firm against all strategies of the devil. For we are not fighting against flesh-and-blood enemies, but against evil rulers and authorities of the unseen world, against mighty powers in this dark world, and against evil spirits in the heavenly places. Therefore, put on every piece of God's armor so you will be able to resist the enemy in the time of evil. Then after the battle you will still be standing firm. Stand your ground, putting on the belt of truth and the body armor of God's righteousness. For shoes, put on the peace that comes from the Good News so that you will be fully prepared. In addition to all of these, hold up the shield of faith to stop the fiery arrows of the devil. Put on salvation as your helmet, and take the sword of the Spirit, which is the word of God. Pray in the Spirit at all times and on every occasion. Stay alert and be persistent in your prayers for all believers everywhere."

7. How can putting on the armor of God plus prayer help you fight the enemy's accusations?

_____

_____

_____

Consider how to implement the following spiritual weapons to fight the Accuser:

Truth _____

God's Righteousness _____

Peace _____

The Gospel _____

Faith _____

Salvation _____

The Holy Spirit _____

The Bible _____

Great work. I hope you are learning that the Accuser has no place in your life. Tell him to "Leave now." In the name of Jesus, he must go. Oh, and he can take his accusations with him. Buh Bye.

The Robber

The Robber is what I'll call the self-talk we use that sounds like "I am (fill in the critical phrase here)." It sounds like first-person self-shaming, wearing down our will to fight for our good, the good of others, and the good of the world day after day.

8. Write down 1 to 2 self-shaming phrases that regularly surface in your self-talk.

For example, "I am ugly" or "I am not smart."

I am _____

I am _____

I am not _____

I am not _____

Way to go identifying Robber phrases. If more come to mind, here is some space to document the thought.

_____

_____

_____

_____

The Robber whispers words that can be used by the enemy to manipulate us and steal our life and joy. Therefore, we need to learn how to recognize and silence the Robber. Everything it says should be challenged and brought up against God's word for a truth check.

2 Timothy 1:7

"For God has not given us a spirit of fear, but of power and of love and of a sound mind."

Usually, the Robber has a few effective sucker punches on repeat. As we ruminate on these hurtful words throughout our lives, we may come to believe them to be un-editable pieces of who we are. As a result, we can feel helpless, ashamed, discouraged, and even depressed.

Robber statements can sabotage our efforts for healthy living when we are attempting positive, difficult change. Here's how: when the Robber drops in our head with a well-oiled critical phrase, such as "I am too old,' it's like a bomb of shame explodes in our brains. This is how the Robber makes fast work of halting important ideas and subsequent changes that would better our lives.

Has the Robber stolen life and joy from you? How?

Explain:

_____

_____

_____

_____

Let's rob the Robber of its ability to steal from us! How? We're going to catch the Robber at work and get rid of it! Scram, Robber!

9. As you go through the day and make healthy choices, notice if the Robber throws out any defeating thoughts that attempt to shame or scare you out of your positive effort to change. Write the phrase(s) down. Notice if the Robber uses some phrases more often than others.

Here's some space to write down the phrases. Taking them out of your head and putting them on paper is the first step toward removal.

1. _____
2. _____
3. _____
4. _____
5. _____

Good job!

Read Romans 8:1

> "Therefore, there is now no condemnation for those who are in Christ Jesus."

10. How can this verse help you fight back against the Robber?

_____
_____
_____
_____

Silencing Negative Self-Talk

Here are practical step-by-step instructions to get rid of the Accuser and the Robber.

1. **Recognize the Accuser and the Robber.**
   - Notice when your inner dialogue includes the Accuser and the Robber.
   - Identify your vulnerable times and emotional states. Does the Robber tend to come around when you are sad? Does the Accuser show up when you are feeling lonely? Angry? Tired? When you're with a parent or a sibling? At a staff meeting?
   - Know ahead of time some of the Accuser's and Robber's favorite lines. Actively replace Accuser and Robber phrases with scripture and positive, uplifting, true statements about yourself.
   - Distinguish between the harsh talk of the Accuser and the Robber versus positive problem-solving inner dialogue.

2. **Refute the Accuser and the Robber.**
   - Tell the Accuser and the Robber the truth and expose the lie. Refute with scripture whenever possible. Jesus was our example in this, as He used scripture to refute the devil when He was tempted in the desert. See Matthew 4:1–10.
   - Don't debate the Accuser or the Robber. Say or read scripture out loud. Memorize scriptures in advance that diffuse phrases the Accuser and the Robber use to control you. Ask God for wisdom and help.

3. **Remove the Accuser and the Robber.**
   - Ask God for protection, help, guidance, and discernment.
   - Tell the Accuser and the Robber to leave by saying "Go away!" or "You're not welcome here. Leave."

- Use a removing fantasy (flush it down the toilet, toss it out the window, flick it off your shoulder, drop kick it ... get rid of that Accuser or Robber). *Don't let the Accuser/Robber travel with you*—they must go now. Turn to God and ask the Holy Spirit to fill the void the Accuser or the Robber has left.

4.   Regain your focus on God's truth and what He has done and is doing in you.

- Consider who God is and that He created you for good works. Remember past victories and good things you're doing now, and acknowledge your abilities, efforts, and successes. Choose to believe God's words, His definition of your worth, and His promises.

5.   Move forward in truth and freedom.

- Take a positive action step that creates life and joy knowing you are loved deeply by God. Ask God what that step could be.

Read Philippians 4:8

> "Finally, brothers and sisters, whatever is true, whatever is noble, whatever is right, whatever is pure, whatever is lovely, whatever is admirable—if anything is excellent or praiseworthy—think about such things."

11. How is Philippians 4:8 a useful guide for replacing Accuser/Robber thoughts?

_____

_____

_____

The Freedom to Forgive Ourselves

As we wrap up this chapter, let's discuss one more reason we say mean things to ourselves: We have not forgiven ourselves for something in our past. Are there things you've done that you can't forgive yourself for? Do you shame yourself over what happened?
Yeah. Me too. Most of us do.
The first step is to ask God for forgiveness.
1 John 1:9
"If we confess our sins, He is faithful and just and will forgive us our sins and purify us from all unrighteousness."
If you haven't already, ask God for forgiveness. You can write a prayer here if you like.

_____

_____

If you've asked for forgiveness, you are forgiven by God! Take a deep breath, thank the Lord, and experience this exciting freedom with Him! He loves you so much.

If you still remind yourself of this failing, are you holding a grudge against yourself that needs to be erased? Write about it here in pencil then erase it, white it out, or cut it out of this book and toss it in the trash. You are forgiven. It's time to move ahead in peace.

_____

_____

Read Colossians 2:12–14

> "For you were buried with Christ when you were baptized. And with Him you were raised to new life because you trusted the mighty power of God, who raised Christ from the dead. You were dead because of your sins and because your sinful nature was not yet cut away. Then God made you alive with Christ, for He forgave all our sins. He canceled the record of the charges against us and took it away by nailing it to the cross."

Picture Jesus canceling that sin, nailing it to the cross with Him, burying it, and raising you to a new life without it. Thank the Lord for wiping this sin clean away and making you new and FREE. Journal your response to the truth and promise written in Colossians and given to you by your loving Savior and faithful friend, Jesus.

12. What can change in your life as you live in freedom from the past?

_____

_____

_____

_____

Combating the Accuser and The Robber with Scripture

Now that you are aware of what the Accuser and the Robber are saying, you can combat their negativity right away with scripture verses. This process and practice of changing thought patterns takes time. That's OK. Keep at it.

Here are some Biblical truths to help you get started fighting the Accuser and the Robber.

1 John 4:4

> "Little children, you are from God and have overcome them, for He who is in you is greater than he who is in the world."

James 4:7

> "Submit yourselves therefore to God. Resist the devil, and he will flee from you."

James 1:5

> "If any of you lacks wisdom, you should ask God, who gives generously to all without finding fault, and it will be given to you."

Proverbs 3:5–6

> "Trust in the Lord with all your heart and lean not on our own understanding. In all your ways acknowledge Him and He will make your path straight."

Ephesians 6:1

> "Put on the whole armor of God, that you may be able to stand against the schemes of the devil."

Matthew 4:10

> "Away from me, Satan! For it is written: 'Worship the Lord your God and serve Him only.'"

Ephesians. 2:10

> "For we are God's masterpiece. He has created us anew in Christ Jesus, so we can do the good things he planned for us long ago."

Philippians 4:8

> "Finally, brothers and sisters, whatever is true, whatever is noble, whatever is right, whatever is pure, whatever is lovely, whatever is admirable—if anything is excellent or praiseworthy—think about such things."

2 Corinthians 12:5

> "We demolish arguments and every pretension that sets itself up against the knowledge of God, and we take captive every thought to make it obedient to Christ."

13. Which of these verses can you start using right way? Explain.

_____

_____

_____

_____

Prepare for Victory

You have everything you need to defeat the Accuser and the Robber. Be prepared and have your defense ready with the *Victory Over Negative Self-Talk* worksheets.

Victory Over Negative Self-Talk

Use this sheet to keep track of Accuser or Robber phrases that come to mind.
1) Write down the phrases exactly as they pop into your head.
2) Next to each phrase, find a Bible Verse you can use to defeat, once and for all, the Accuser and the Robber.

Wisdom from the Word:

"For the word of God is living and effective and sharper than any double-edged sword, penetrating as far as the separation of soul and spirit, joints and marrow. It is able to judge the ideas and thoughts of the heart."

Hebrews 4:12 HCSB

Accuser/Robber phrase:

....
....
....
....

Scripture I can use to demolish the thought:

....
....
....
....

Accuser/Robber phrase:

....
....
....
....

Scripture I can use to demolish the thought:

....
....
....
....

Accuser/Robber phrase:

....
....
....
....

Scripture I can use to demolish the thought:

....
....
....
....

Victory Over Negative Self-Talk Continued....

Wisdom from the Word:

"We demolish arguments and every pretension that sets itself up against the knowledge of God, and we take captive every thought to make it obedient to Christ."

2 Corinthians 12:5

Accuser/Robber phrase:

Scripture I can use to demolish the thought:

Accuser/Robber phrase:

Scripture I can use to demolish the thought:

Accuser/Robber phrase:

Scripture I can use to demolish the thought:

Accuser/Robber phrase:

Scripture I can use to demolish the thought:

14. What is one thing you can do to apply what you learned in this chapter starting today?

_____

_____

_____

_____

Promise Prompt:

Cut this verse out and post it in a place you visit often to remind you that God is helping you overcome unhealthy eating.

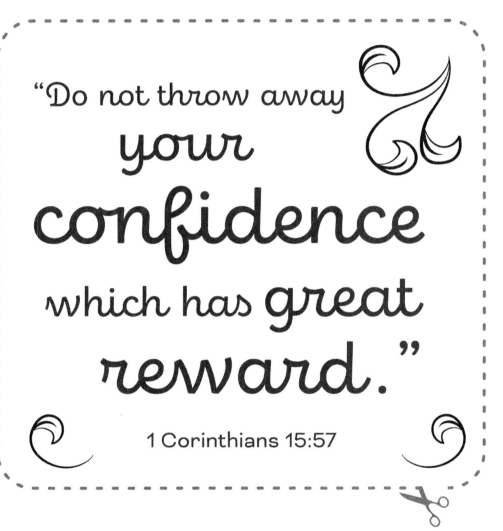

"Do not throw away your confidence which has great reward."

1 Corinthians 15:57

Journal Your Thoughts

Here is more space to write.

Date: ....

I am thankful for: ....

Take a "Victory Lap!"

Celebrate success big or small!

Victory Lap: Pause to celebrate your win. Thank the Lord and tell yourself you did a good thing.
Smile and approve of the progress you are making. Enjoy how good it feels. Well done. You did it!!

Date: ....

Victory: ....

How I feel about myself: ....

Why I did it:
....
....
....

Things that helped me succeed:
....
....
....

How God helped me:
....
....

I have new hope that: ....
....

I could try this strategy again for another win:
....

What I have learned from the victory:
....
....

I am thankful for: ....
....

Chapter 6

I Think My Wheel Of Life Has A Flat

What we'll talk about:

How our current circumstances might be triggering overeating.

Why it matters:

Jesus has the power (not food) to satisfy our souls.

Wisdom from the Word:

"He has satisfied the thirsty soul, and the hungry soul He has filled with what is good."

Psalm 107:8–9

Recommended Song of Preparation:

"Evidence" by Josh Baldwin

Share a success story about applying Chapter 5 to your life.

_____

_____

_____

_____

Awesome!

Why Yes, I Am Hungry

Full disclosure: I'm hungry a lot. In fact, if you caught me alone during the day, you might hear me say to my stomach, "I know you're hungry. You're always hungry," and "Hello tummy, it's not all about you today."

You might be able to relate when I say I can eat when it's time to eat _and_ when it's not time to eat, when I'm hungry and when I'm not hungry ... _and_ eat some more. I could graze or pound a plate of goodies all.day.long.

For those of us who love food, we munch for many reasons, physical hunger being one ... but there are countless other reasons to consume food that have absolutely nothing to do with nutrition or hunger. We find ourselves asking questions like:

"Why do I eat so much extra and/or unhealthy food _even though I want to stop_?"

"Why is eating such a knee-jerk reaction?" and

"How did I end up binging _again_?"

The answers to these questions are as individual as the person searching for solutions, yet there are common recovery options we can explore together.

The Meal that Isn't Just a Meal

Every meal or snack drops like a parachuter into our life's current state of affairs. It may fall on a peaceful meadow, a celebratory party, or a war zone. Due to the complex and fast-paced nature of daily living (be it the places, players, or problems), we may or may not know exactly why we are eating. All we know is that we _need to eat_. To learn how to stop unhealthy eating patterns, a precious gift we can give ourselves is _time_—time to consider our current situation and learn how our circumstances may be affecting our food consumption.

For example: In one instance, you might know exactly why you're eating. It's 6:00 p.m., time for dinner, and the family is sitting around the table. Let's eat!

Yet, dinner may _also_ be layered with emotions due to an insensitive statement made by your spouse, roommate, or teenager. When you are hurt, disappointed, and facing a pile of dishes, suddenly, one portion isn't enough. A reasonable dinner must now be chased with leftover french fries dipped in ice cream. "Yes," we tell ourselves, "that would taste really good right now." In other words, that would be just the "soft landing" needed in this emotional war zone.

On the other hand, dinner might be a festive occasion! Maybe you completed a demanding project at work, and it's time to party. Celebration is a common reason to justify overeating. Celebrations are very often complicated with lesser acknowledged, difficult emotions. Combine joy and "deserving" a reward with things like:

social anxiety
family togetherness
stress about tomorrow
guilty feelings for overeating

Voila! What was a party turns into a field of emotional landmines that catapult us into food oblivion.

Land With Power

Whatever your food terrain, the sneak-attack nature of emotional eating is at times evident. Other times it is buried under a messy pile of emotional dirty laundry that we're too busy to sort.

Yet, you can learn to land in any situation like a champion. You know the stance I mean! Whenever a hero falls out of the sky and lands on the ground, they crouch on one knee, fist to the ground, head up, in a proactive, ready for anything, mental and physical position of power and strength. We can take this visual model of readiness into our eating events.

But how? Like any hero, you're going to need some time in the tactical room with your commander and chief (Jesus) to examine the landscape, prepare in advance, and get your instructions. Exploring our current life conditions can help us identify food danger zones. When we understand what exactly we are facing, we more clearly see what situations are causing the emotions that push us to eat outside our healthy eating plan. Let's look closer and identify potential food danger zones using the **Wheel of Life**.

The Wheel of Life

The **Wheel of Life** is a circle divided into pie-shaped pieces, each representing a part of life that affects your feelings of well-being. We'll break down the following categories of your life landscape and rate your *current* satisfaction with each area.

Physical Environment—Your current living situation.

Family Life—Your family relationships and how they might be affecting your satisfaction with life.

Spiritual Well-being—Your spiritual growth, church life, and your relationship with God.

Mental Health—Your current mental well-being and mental health. This may mean an actual diagnosis but includes a mental state such as stressed, joyful, afraid, or burdened.

Friendships—Your current friendships.

Personal Development—Your satisfaction with your current state of personal growth, such as education. Personal development may also incorporate a wide variety of learning opportunities and avenues, such as learning a language online or listening to informative podcasts for example.

Love and Relationships—Your romantic relationships and/or marriage.

Physical Health—Your satisfaction with the physical health of your body.

Fun, Hobbies, and Recreation—Your satisfaction regarding opportunities to do pleasurable activities just for fun.

Money and Finances—Your financial situation, including but not limited to savings, earnings, debt, spending cash, etc.

Career and Job—What you do for work. You may be a court reporter, caregiver, parent, or cook. "Career and Job" doesn't necessarily imply compensation; parenting is full-time work without a paycheck.

Instructions: Note the numbers radiating out from 1-10 corresponding to each category on the wheel. Fill out the wheel by circling the level of satisfaction you feel with each. One being very low satisfaction and 10 the highest level of satisfaction. Rate the categories on how you feel today. When you have circled a number for each category, connect the circles or dots you've drawn around the numbers. Notice where your **Wheel of Life** "pie" dips toward the center. These are the areas you are less satisfied with at the moment. It's perfectly normal to see "dips" in satisfaction. I don't know anyone whose **Wheel of Life** is perfectly rounded all the time. In fact, there can be many good reasons for a lower satisfaction rating. For example, we may be focusing on our family, and thus our job satisfaction is lower. We may be paying for school, and as a result, "Personal Development" ranks higher, but "Money and Finances" dips lower due to the expenses tied to education.

> **Personal Variations:** Try not to compare your wheel ratings to someone else's. Each person defines the value of the numbers a little differently, and each person is in a different life circumstance. The point is to have a visual representation of *your* areas of higher and lower satisfaction right now.

> Are you ready?
> Let's fill out your **Wheel of Life**. [1]

---

[1] The Wheel of Life is credited to Paul J. Meyer and the Wellness Wheel to Dr. Bill Hettler. I have adapted the concepts for the purposes of this material.

Wheel of Life

Rate your level of satisfaction in each area of your life. 1 is low satisfaction, 10 being highest.
Once you have marked each number, connect each number forming a new outer edge for your circle.

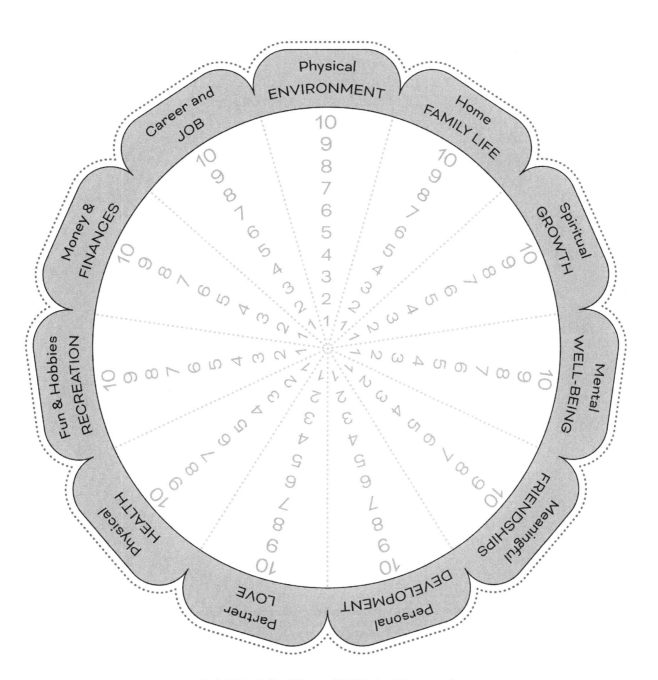

1. Examine your **Wheel of Life** result. Write down what stands out to you.

_____
_____
_____
_____
_____
_____
_____

2. What are some of your high scores?

_____
_____
_____
_____
_____
_____
_____

3. What area could you invest in that would positively affect the increase of other areas? Explain.

_____
_____
_____
_____
_____
_____
_____

4. Write about the feelings that came up while you worked on your **Wheel of Life**. Explain why you think these surfaced.

Example:
Feeling: fear
Why you think it surfaced: I might never get married

Feeling: _____
Why you think it surfaced: _____

Feeling: _____
Why you think it surfaced: _____

Feeling: _____
Why you think it surfaced: _____

_____

5. Do any of these feelings associated with life circumstances drive you to eat unhealthy food for comfort, eat when you are not hungry, and/or overeat? Describe:

_____

_____

_____

_____

_____

_____

_____

_____

_____

6. How does food *help you* when you need comfort in a tough life situation? How does eating food for comfort *hurt you*?

Help:

_____

_____

_____

_____

_____

_____

_____

Hurt:

_____

_____

_____

_____

_____

_____

_____

7. How can an awareness of these results help you to "land" with strength?

_____

_____

_____

_____

_____

_____

_____

Pumping up Your Wheel of Life

It's easy to believe the lie that eating unhealthy food in unhealthy ways improves quality of life. The truth is: eating can't fix a flat on the **Wheel of Life**. Food can fill a stomach, but it can't actually make life improvements or fill a void in the soul.

8. Food can't increase your **Wheel of Life** ratings (move us from a 4 → 5 → 6). Choose a category you rated lower on your Wheel. What small *action* (besides eating) will make you feel better AND pump up this category on your **Wheel of life**?

_____
_____
_____
_____
_____
_____
_____

Oswald Chambers said, "There is only One Being who can satisfy the last aching abyss of the human heart, and that is the Lord Jesus Christ."

Psalm 107:8–9 says:

> "Let them give thanks to the Lord for His faithful love and his wondrous works for all humanity! (Holman Christian Standard Bible)
> For He satisfies the thirsty soul and fills the hungry soul with what is good."
> (New American Standard Bible)

9. God alone has the power to satisfy our soul. *Food does not have that power.* How can (and does) the Lord satisfy you when life leaves you "hungry"?

_____
_____
_____
_____
_____
_____
_____

10. When you stop eating for satisfaction, what can you do to connect with the Lord for fulfillment? For example, play praise music and sing along, write in a journal, etc.

_____
_____
_____
_____
_____
_____
_____

11. How can you catch yourself eating for relief and go to God for comfort instead?

_____
_____
_____
_____
_____
_____

12. Write about a time when an area you ranked higher in satisfaction was once lower. Describe the process of transitioning from low satisfaction to high. How long did it take? What changed? What role did you play in the change? What role did God play in the increase?

_____

_____

_____

_____

_____

_____

_____

_____

_____

_____

_____

_____

13. How does remembering this story give you hope for the areas that are currently ranked lower in satisfaction?

_____

_____

_____

_____

_____

_____

_____

_____

_____

_____

_____

14. How might remembering God's power, goodness, and faithfulness in the past help you allow Him to satisfy your needs in the future?

_____

_____

_____

_____

_____

_____

Chapter 6 Wrap-Up

15. Thank God for the areas in your life that you are happy with! Write down blessings you are experiencing right now.

_____   _____
_____   _____
_____   _____
_____   _____
_____   _____

16. What is one thing you can do to apply what you learned in this chapter starting today?

_____
_____
_____
_____
_____
_____
_____
_____
_____
_____
_____

Promise Prompt:

Cut this verse out and post it in a place you visit often to remind you that God is helping you overcome unhealthy eating.

"He has satisfied the thirsty soul, And the hungry soul He has filled with what is good."

Psalm 107:9

Journal Your Thoughts

Here is more space to write.

Date: ....

....

....

....

....

....

....

....

....

I am thankful for: ....

....

....

Take a "Victory Lap!"

Celebrate success big or small!

Victory Lap: Pause to celebrate your win. Thank the Lord and tell yourself you did a good thing.
Smile and approve of the progress you are making. Enjoy how good it feels. Well done. You did it!!

Date: ....

Victory: ....

How I feel about myself: ....

Why I did it:
....
....
....

Things that helped me succeed:
....
....
....

How God helped me:
....
....

I have new hope that: ....
....

I could try this strategy again for another win:
....
....

What I have learned from the victory:
....
....

I am thankful for: ....
....
....

Chapter 7

Bring More Peanut Butter, I Need To Fill A Crack In My Heart

What we'll talk about:

Why we use food to fix our hurts.

Why it matters:

The power to fix and heal comes from Christ alone.

Wisdom from the Word:

"Peace I leave with you; my peace I give you. I do not give to you as the world gives. Do not let your hearts be troubled and do not be afraid."

John 14:27

Recommended Song of Preparation:

"It is Well" by Bethel Music

Share a success story about applying Chapter 6 to your life.

_____

_____

_____

_____

Way to go!

Krinkle Cut Chips... Take Me Away!

A year into my second go in a food addiction program I had a handle on what foods to avoid until I was stronger. One of the foods on my list was chips because I have a record of not eating just one but *one-fifty.*

We found ourselves at the dining room table talking with family about holiday plans and I began to stress about planning food for the holidays, eating food during the holidays and maintaining my weight loss over the holidays. Before any of us knew what was happening, the chip bowl was empty.

Oddly, the entire party size bowl of chips did not make my uncomfortable feelings go away or help me communicate my needs to the family around the table. Maybe the crumbs would do the trick. "No," I thought to myself, "I can't lick salt off the bottom of a chip bowl in front of people."

Hm. Maybe if I shook the bowl really hard over my paper plate no one would notice.

And then, I caught myself believing a couple of lies. Maybe you can relate. 1) If I eat the (chips) the bad feelings will go away. 2) If I eat the (chips) I can avoid communicating my needs 3) If I eat the (chips) the problem will disappear, and I won't need to face it and figure out how to resolve it. Conclusion: food, in this case (chips) will fix all my food and family problems.

Turns out, stuffing food in my face didn't make the situation go away, and it certainly didn't fix the problems. In fact, food compromised me by a) making it difficult for me to talk because I was eating and focused on food b) making it look like in truth I don't care about what I put in my body and c) making me feel so bad about myself I didn't feel worthy to speak up.

My feelings were attached to eating food and I couldn't separate food from fear *and* know what to do with fear and the root cause of the fear if chips were on the table.

In that moment, I looked to chips to save me from uncomfortable feelings. I learned a very important lesson: there aren't enough chips in the world to solve challenging family conversations or fix Thanksgiving dinner for ten.

Why Trust Jesus?

Jesus told us we could trust Him. Why? Because HE is the one with ALL the power. Check this out:

Jesus said in Matthew 28:18, "All authority (all power and absolute rule) in heaven, and on earth, has been given to me."

Wait, what did that say? Some authority on earth, all in heaven? Some in heaven and some on earth? Nope. It says ALL. ALL OF IT. ALL power, all the time, over everything.

Let's pause for a moment and ask ourselves if we are allowing food to interfere with the power Jesus might display in our lives. Proverbs 3:5 says, "Trust the Lord with all your heart." There are moments, days, weeks, and even years that this can be a real challenge. However, seeing the world through the truth lens of who Jesus is and how powerful He is can help.

How does knowing that Jesus is the One with the power and we are His help you gain perspective and peace concerning something in your life that is troubling you right now?

1. What is troubling you?

    _____
    _____
    _____
    _____

2. How do Jesus' words about having all the power add perspective to your concerns?

    _____
    _____
    _____
    _____

There are wonderful moments in this life, hard ones too. None of us get off this planet unscathed and unscarred. The many emotions, including uncomfortable feelings, are an inextricable part of daily life and worthy of attention and care. For those of us who love food, eating can be a deeply personal way of acting on, without facing, formidable and painful hurts.

When we "eat away" our problems in search of peace, we hand over the peace Jesus can give in exchange for the short-term "peace" food gives. Really short term. Sometimes, it's only seconds. Oh man, it's a bummer when that happens. Can you relate?

Kind of like gambling at a slot machine … maybe this time, the food will give me the peace I need; maybe I just need more food … come onnnnnn chocolate …

3. Talk about a time you chose to go to food for peace, and peace didn't last very long at all. In fact, you may have gone back for more in hopes of better satisfaction.

    _____
    _____
    _____
    _____

Next, to reassure ourselves eating for peace is "fine" (even though we know in our heart it's not working), we shrug it off because it makes us feel better, and we tell ourselves, "My eating isn't hurting anyone."

Overeating IS hurting someone. It's hurting *you*.

Ouch, I know, that stung me a little too.

I have something sensitive to share with you. I don't want to hurt food's feelings, so we may ask it to leave the room.

"Food, please wait outside for a moment."
(Is it gone? Ok, here we go …)

(Whisper voice) *Food can't fix life's problems.*

(Gasp! I know. Food would be so insulted right now.)

Food is an inanimate object, and as important as it can be in our lives, it only acts as fuel for our body—no more, no less. It has no magical powers. The truth is: food can't *"make it better."* That's just smoke and mirrors with a side of hash browns.

Don't get me wrong, food can be a good thing. We need it for survival. But Satan has been using food for a long time to get people to sin. Consider Eve and the first sin in the garden of Eden. I mean, if the devil got Eve with a piece of fruit, imagine what he can do with a pint of Dulce de Leche.

Kidding aside, our enemy and his spiritual forces of evil are not above using something good to take you out. He will use food to destroy you if that's what it takes. He'll even help you justify it. Maybe it sounds like, "Well, I don't do crack cocaine, pot, or porn; another fudgie bar isn't so bad. After all, food is necessary for life."

If said fudgie bar (or another unhealthy or excessive food choice) is making us feel better and "giving us peace," *we're not getting peace and power from Jesus.* The Bible doesn't say food has the power; Jesus says *He has all the power.*

Let's investigate where using food for peace may have started and how certain thought processes may still be functioning in our lives today.

4. Write about the first time you remember being given food or eating food to "make it better."

_____
_____
_____
_____

5. Write about your current "food will fix it" eating behavior.

_____
_____
_____
_____

6. What specific food(s) are you using right now to "make it better"? (Name the exact food or ingredient. For example, mint chip ice cream or pretzels.) Be specific. For example, instead of "chocolate," write the name or form of chocolate. Instead of carbs, write "tortillas."

_____
_____
_____
_____

7. Fill in the following sentences. Example:

When I <u>wake up,</u> I want <u>hazelnut creamer</u> in my coffee because <u>I hate mornings.</u>

When I <u>get my grandkids,</u> I <u>want to go to ice cream</u> because <u>I want them to love being with me.</u>

When I _____, I want _____ because
_____.

When I _____, I want _____ because
_____.

Good job.

It can be difficult to isolate what we are eating and why specifically. How often do we really pause to consider the emotions attached to specific foods? In fact, let's do a little more of that self-study right now.

Identify Your "Food Drivers"

Feelings can cause cravings. Therefore, it's important to think about what feelings are taking over the wheel in our car of life and driving us straight into the arms of unhealthy food. I call these feelings "Food Drivers." As you read the following list of feelings or Food Drivers:

1) **Circle** the feelings you experience that really bother you. None of the feelings are pleasant, so we're going to focus on circling the ones that are particularly disruptive to your mental state of well-being.
2) **Add a star** next to an emotion if it ignites a hunger pang, acid reflux, food craving, or other food or stomach physical response when you read the word.

Extra credit: If you read an emotion and the word ignites a food craving, and a specific food comes to mind, write the name of the food next to the word.

Feeling hungry just thinking about reading a list of uncomfortable feelings?

Extra, extra credit for powering through anyway! You can do this!

Bottom line: Do you associate any of the feelings on the list with eating and/or specific foods?

Example from my own life:

Reading the word *abandoned*, I feel my body tense up.

Circle the word "abandoned."

Reading the word *abandoned* makes me need to taste something.

Add a star next to "abandoned."

Suddenly I am feeling a little desperate for crunchy salt and vinegar chips.

Write salt and vinegar chips next to "abandoned."

Sometimes while filling out this sheet, we realize that we may have some life challenges that are bigger hills than we know how to climb. It's okay. Life can be unexpected and really hard. Pray about what finding healthy support might look like for you. God can, and often does, use others to help us grow and thrive through challenges. Make a list of three people you can call if you need to talk to someone after completing this exercise.

1._____
2._____
3._____

This may bring up some hurt. It may reveal some pains you aren't sure you're ready to face.
But you can do this, and it will help you identify foods that are taking the place of Jesus' peace and power in your life.

Take your time; this exercise is not easy.

Find a quiet place.

Pray before you begin.

Ready? Let's go.

Psalm 139:1–10

"You have searched me, Lord,
and you know me.

You know when I sit and when I rise;
you perceive my thoughts from afar.

You discern my going out and my lying down;
you are familiar with all my ways.

Before a word is on my tongue
you, Lord, know it completely.

You hem me in behind and before,
and you lay your hand upon me.

Such knowledge is too wonderful for me,
too lofty for me to attain.

Where can I go from your Spirit?
Where can I flee from your presence?

If I go up to the heavens, you are there;
if I make my bed in the depths, you are there.

If I rise on the wings of the dawn,
if I settle on the far side of the sea,

even there your hand will guide me,
your right hand will hold me fast."

Emotional Eating "Food Drivers"

Below is a list of emotions that may be driving you to eat unhealthy food, or eat food in an unhealthy way. There is a space next to the emotion to write any cravings or feelings you may have when you read the word. Write down what comes to mind.

DISQUIET FEELING/CRAVING
afraid
dread
anxiety
scared
worried
mistrustful
panicky
suspicious
concerned
forboding
startled
cluttered
agitated
uncomfortable
unnerved
unsettled
distressed
irritable
jittery
stressed out

UPSET FEELING/CRAVING
impatient
exasperated
irritated
shocked
unhappy
uneasy
dissatisfied
annoyed
angry
irate
chaotic
overwrought
turbulent
outraged
perturbed
bitter
resentful
contempt
hate
horror
hostility
repulsion
frazzled

TIRED FEELING/CRAVING
burned out
exhausted
depleted
weary
worn down
beat
fatigue
fried
consumed
broken down
overwhelmed
wasted
lethargic

EMBARASSED FEELING/CRAVING
ashamed
distraught
distressed
humiliated
regretful
sorry
demeaned
flustered
guilty
mortified
self-conscious
flustered

Emotional Eating
"Food Drivers"

SAD
FEELING/CRAVING

disappointed
rejected
hopeless
wretched
disheartened
forlorn
melancholy
abandoned
despondent
bitter
tearful
despairing
dismal
inconsolable
bereaved
distraught
yearning
jealous
nostalgic
pining

HURT
FEELING/CRAVING

pain
agony
devastation
miserable
remorseful
distress
tortured
desperate
jealous

AMBIVALENT
FEELING/CRAVING

confused
hesitant
lost
perplexed
torn
baffled
rattled
surprised
reeling
mystified
restless

ALONE
FEELING/CRAVING

disconnected
apathetic
bored
cold
distant
distracted
numb
indifferent
isolated
betrayed
grief
heartbroken
dejected
forlorn
vulnerable
fragile
insecure
sensitive
helpless

OTHER
FEELING/CRAVING

NOTES

Great work!
Let's examine your results.

8. What foods are you craving and/or eating to soothe uncomfortable and/or painful emotions?

_____
_____
_____
_____
_____
_____

9. Which (if any) emotions do you attach to foods you regularly consume? Example: "When I am stressed, I need something crunchy like chips."

_____
_____
_____
_____
_____
_____

10. Describe when you are particularly vulnerable to unhealthy eating behaviors.

_____
_____
_____
_____
_____
_____

This is a conundrum because, if we're honest, the food does make us feel better short term, and as a result, we have come to rely on certain foods for relief. While food can help emotions and pain for a time, it **cannot heal** them.

11. Tell a story about a time you relied on food to fix an uncomfortable feeling or situation and food didn't fix it. For example, I ate a pint of ice cream every night for a week after I lost my job.

_____
_____
_____
_____
_____
_____

12. What have you learned from your own life experience about "eating to solve problems"?

_____
_____
_____
_____

13. Do we want to be *helped*, or do we want to be *healed*? To what end are we using food … and can it live up to that expectation? Journal your thoughts.

_____
_____
_____
_____
_____

14. Let's pause and connect with the Lord. Tell the Lord about how food helps you in your pain and joys. Ask Him how you can move forward in a new way, connecting to Jesus and asking for His power to help **and** heal.

_____
_____
_____
_____
_____

Well done. This can be a difficult exercise. You did it!

The Freedom to Feel

For many who struggle with overeating, somewhere along the line, we were told to "sit down and shut up" when it came to expressing our emotions. Maybe we were ignored. It's possible someone listened but pretended like the conversation never happened. Some parents gave us food with the implication, "Eat this and go away." We may have been dismissed with a wave of the hand or told statements like "You're too much," or "children are to be seen and not heard." However it happened, whether once or a hundred times, our feelings and needs were diminished, insulted, or ignored. "Stop crying, or I'll give you something to cry about," and being treated like a waste of space caused us to believe expressing emotions was at best useless and at worst unsafe or even dangerous.

15. Talk about a time your feelings were diminished, ridiculed, or ignored.

_____
_____
_____
_____
_____

16. How does this event affect the way you express emotions today?

_____
_____
_____
_____
_____

17. Would you rather eat than express feelings? Describe.

_____
_____
_____
_____
_____
_____

18. List emotions you feel safe expressing freely.

_____   _____
_____   _____
_____   _____

19. Explain.

_____
_____
_____
_____
_____
_____

20. List emotions you *do not* feel comfortable expressing freely.

_____   _____
_____   _____
_____   _____

21. Pick one emotion from question 20. Write about why you do not feel comfortable expressing it freely.

_____
_____
_____
_____
_____
_____

22. Describe a painful emotion you often strive to overcome: _____

23. How much food is it going to take, for how long, to make this emotion go away? What is the result of using food to overcome this painful feeling in your life?

_____
_____
_____
_____
_____
_____

God Is a Good Listener

The good news for those of us who have been hurt in this way is this: God listens, God cares, and we can share with Him the whole truth about what we are going through.

Psalm 56:8 says:

> "You keep track of all my sorrows. You have collected all my tears in your bottle. You
> have recorded each one in your book."

24. What are you experiencing currently that you need God to care about?

_____
_____
_____
_____

25. What does this verse tell you about how the Lord cares about your life hurts? How does knowing this encourage you to talk to Him about the emotions you are facing?

_____
_____
_____
_____

26. List some practical ways you can remind yourself to go to God to listen, help, and give you peace.

_____
_____
_____
_____

27. Ask God for ideas concerning how to safely express emotions without eating in an unhealthy way. List any ideas that come to mind.

_____
_____
_____
_____
_____

Seeking and Finding True Peace

John 14:27 says:

> "Peace I leave with you; my peace I give you. I do not give to you as the world gives.
> Do not let your hearts be troubled and do not be afraid."

Not only will God give us more power and more healing than food, but God will also give us more *peace* than food can every single time. Let's explore the difference between going to God for peace and help versus going to food for peace and help.

28. Compare and contrast how food *helps* you versus how God *helps* you.

Food Name	Help Food Gives	Help God Gives

Compare and contrast the *peace* food gives versus the *peace* God gives.

Food Name	Peace Food Gives	Help God Gives

29. What stands out to you specifically about the difference between what food can do versus God's sovereignty and power?

_____
_____
_____
_____
_____
_____

The Lord loves you so much. As you release food and cling to Him more each day, you will discover just how deep His powerful, life-changing love can be for *you.*

This chapter was not easy, but you did it. You have made many discoveries concerning how intricately your feelings are tied to the desire for and consumption of food. Great job!

Chapter 7 Wrap-Up

30. What is one thing you can do to apply what you learned in this chapter starting today?

_____
_____
_____
_____

Promise Prompt:
Cut this verse out and post it in a place you visit often to remind you that God is helping you overcome unhealthy eating.

"*Peace*
I leave with you;
my peace I give you.
I do not give to you
as the world gives.
Do not let
your hearts be troubled and
do not be afraid."

John 14:27

Journal Your Thoughts

Here is more space to write.

Date: ....

....
....
....
....
....
....
....
....

I am thankful for: ....
....
....

Take a "Victory Lap!"

Celebrate success big or small!

Victory Lap: Pause to celebrate your win. Thank the Lord and tell yourself you did a good thing.
Smile and approve of the progress you are making. Enjoy how good it feels. Well done. You did it!!

Date: ....

Victory: ....

How I feel about myself: ....

Why I did it:
....
....
....
....

Things that helped me succeed:
....
....
....

How God helped me:
....
....

I have new hope that: ....
....

I could try this strategy again for another win:
....

What I have learned from the victory:
....
....

I am thankful for: ....
....

Chapter 8

There's A God-Shaped Hole In All Of Us.
Mine Is Roughly The Size Of An Apple Fritter.

What we'll talk about:

How we put food on the throne of our life as savior and friend ... crowding out Jesus.

Why it matters:

Jesus is the only Savior.

Wisdom from the Word:

Thou shalt have no other gods before me."

Exodus 20:3

Recommended Song of Preparation:

"First" by Lauren Daigle

Share a success story about applying Chapter 7 to your life.

_____

_____

_____

_____

Way to Go!

Step Aside Food, There's a Real Savior in Town

Intentionally detaching food from our feelings and putting food in its place as an inanimate object, not an active helper (which is the job of the Creator, not the created), takes effort and practice. It also requires discernment and carving out time to think about why *exactly* we are eating.

Well done, YOU, for putting in the work and prayers to make these important adjustments in your life. This is definitely worth a victory lap!

You may still long for food. It's easy to romanticize what food was when it was good to us and forget the dark side of unhealthy eating. Oh, the lies we have believed about overeating and junk food! It's a form of seduction we've given in to, and it's tough to break free. Who hasn't been wooed by a silky, sweet fudge sundae at least once?

At the core of our romance with food, we thought food was a friend who could turn around bad days, heal a hurt heart, calm stress, and more. Maybe, the truth is, food has been a friend … and for a time, it was a good friend.

Truthfully, food has helped me survive difficulties. An everyday story from my life is how food aided my survival during the "the bewitching hour." This is the block of the day after school and before dinner when the kids are doing homework. They are run down, cranky, hungry, and demanding. Amid it all, I need to clean, make dinner, explain math that may as well be a foreign language, and referee arguments without a flag, instant replay, or cooler of Gatorade to dump on the winner. Will someone please get me some noise-canceling headphones and a bag of chocolate chips? During intense survival moments like the bewitching hour, it's hard to stop and pray before pouring ranch dressing on pizza … not to mention times of life that are far more painful to endure.

1. Tell a story of survival from your life when God brought you through.

_____

_____

_____

_____

_____

2. Write about how food helped you through this tough time.

_____

_____

_____

_____

_____

Who's on First?

When food is our first choice to comfort ourselves, problem solve, and celebrate, it follows that in some way, deep inside, we are letting food creep in to "save the day." This means food gets to be the substitute hero before giving the real Champion, our Lord, the opportunity to save us *for real*.

When we depend on food to survive problems or see us through difficult moments, *we are crowding out Jesus.* God wants to be the one we depend on. He loves us, and He cares about our hearts. He died for us, after all. Greater love has no man (or chili dog) than this. ("Chili dog" added by author.)

John 15:13 says:

> "Greater love has no one than this: to lay down one's life for one's friends."

Read Exodus 20:3:

> "Thou shalt have no other gods before me."

This verse means exactly what it says—our hearts must allow no other person, place, or thing *before* God. God is first, *or* the thing we are putting first is first.

If we go to food *first* to celebrate or problem solve, we are choosing a *thing* before Him. God is not going to make us love Him or control our desire to go to Him. Choosing Him first (or not first) is up to us.

In this world where burgers are king, and every craving can be met in minutes, it takes an intentional effort on our part to make Jesus the King. This means He is our first choice as friend, our first choice as provider, our first choice as helper, and our first love. The painful truth is going to anything before we go to God is idolatry. I know that sounds harsh but let that sink in for a moment. The thing we choose to put before God is an idol. Yes, sadly, even a bowl of peanut butter pretzel bites.

Food has a habit of sneaking into first place, and sometimes it's so subtle. If we are not alert, it's easy to miss the bait and switch. How many times do we eat believing food will "help us"? For example:

"Ugh, why does my sister always have to make this my responsibility? I'll get drive-thru. Fries always calm me down."

"I just want to sit in front of the TV, eat chips and popcorn, and not think about what happened at work today. Then I'll feel better."

"I passed the test! Time for cake!"

"My teenager is so mean! I need help dealing with her attitude. But first a candy bar."

"I'm so lonely and eating chocolate before bed cheers me up."

"I am disappointed. At this point, what's another cookie?"

I'm not saying that it's wrong to eat these foods or that a person shouldn't celebrate with food or eat fun food now and again. The point is when we have a need, either food or Jesus will be our first go-to. We can't have both God and food playing the role of savior. There is one Savior. Who will it be?

Put an X next to the name of your Savior.
____ Jesus   ____ Food

I think you probably put an X next to Jesus. I hope you did! But even when we know Jesus is the true Savior, we can still go to food first for comfort.

3.   Share a story about a time you went to food for comfort before going to God for comfort?

_____
_____
_____
_____
_____
_____

4.   Ask God to reveal lies you have believed about the power of food. Write what comes to mind. Example: "It doesn't matter what I eat" or "fries will get me through this."

_____
_____
_____
_____
_____
_____

Pray about the following and journal what comes to mind.

5.   What false teaching have I believed about how unhealthy food can make my life better? (If you have trouble thinking of one, just look at a fast-food billboard on your way to work.)

_____
_____
_____
_____
_____
_____

6.   What beliefs do I have about food helping soothe fear and anxiety?

_____
_____
_____
_____
_____
_____

7. What beliefs do I have about food helping disappointment and sadness?

_____
_____
_____
_____
_____

8. How might shame and food be connected in my life?

_____
_____
_____
_____
_____

9. How are love and food connected in my life?

_____
_____
_____
_____
_____

10. When do I deserve unhealthy food? Why do I believe this?

_____
_____
_____
_____
_____

11. How might pride and food be connected in my life?

_____
_____
_____
_____
_____

Good job! That's some deep and powerful work. Bravo!!

Jesus Is the Source of Power

We all need to eat. What we're learning is that as long as we have food on the throne of our life, expecting it to do what only God can, *we are denying Jesus the opportunity to do what only HE can do.* If food is first, we're putting the real power second. Yikes. I don't know about you, but I want the true power in first place, pronto.

In John 15:5 Jesus says,

> "I am the vine; you are the branches.
> If you remain in me and I in you, you will bear much fruit.
> apart from me you can do nothing."

When we connect to Jesus first, we are connecting to the vine, aka "the power." Food may be energy, but Jesus is power. There are only two options. Either we connect to the true vine (Jesus), and we bear much fruit, or we connect to another vine (like food) and can do nothing. There isn't a world where misused food helps us. It's Jesus or nothing.

Let's take food off the throne and invite Jesus back, shall we?

Read 1 John 1:9:

> "If we confess our sins, He is faithful and just and will forgive us our sins and purify us
> from all unrighteousness."

Ask for help and forgiveness as the Lord guides you. Pray for wisdom to know how to put God on the throne of your life instead of food.

Pray with me:

Dear Lord,
I want to remove food from the throne of my life as my first choice as friend and savior. I choose you first, Jesus. Please take Your place as the rightful Lord, Savior, and Friend in my life. Please help me connect to You, the true vine. I ask You to help me with my day-to-day needs and struggles in a way only You can: to save, help redeem, restore, and give unspeakable joy and peace. I love You, Jesus. Thank You for loving me. I'm sorry I have gone to food for help first. Please forgive me and remind me that You alone are my refuge and strength and ever-present help in trouble. Amen.

12. Write any thoughts that come to mind after praying this prayer.

_____
_____
_____
_____

Well done!

Next, let's talk about finding soul satisfaction even if our tongues and tummies aren't as happy and full as they want to be. (They can really act like the center of the universe sometimes!)

Bread for the Soul

Read Matthew 4:4:

> "But He (Jesus) answered and said, it is written, 'Man shall not live by bread alone, but
> on every word that comes from the mouth of God.'"

Read Psalm 73:26:

> "My flesh and my heart may fail, but God is the strength of my heart and my portion forever."

13. What do these verses mean to you when applied to your eating habits?

_____
_____
_____
_____
_____
_____

There is more to life than food. As we consider how satisfying the Lord is and prioritize Him over food, it can be scary. To help us do that, let's remember His past faithfulness to bolster our ability to trust Him with our future.

14. What has God done in the past to help you overcome a significant personal challenge?

_____
_____
_____
_____
_____

15. What does this tell you about:

a. God's character?

_____
_____
_____
_____

b. How God feels about you?

_____
_____
_____
_____
_____

c. God's desire to help you overcome your food challenges?

_____
_____
_____
_____
_____

Write a prayer thanking God for all He has done in the past and ask Him to help you with your present and your future.

_____

_____

_____

_____

Great job taking food off the throne of your life! Now, let's keep it off.

Chapter 8 Wrap-Up

16. What is one thing you can do to apply what you learned in this chapter starting today?

_____

_____

_____

_____

Promise Prompt:

Cut this verse out and post it in a place you visit often to remind you that God is helping you overcome unhealthy eating.

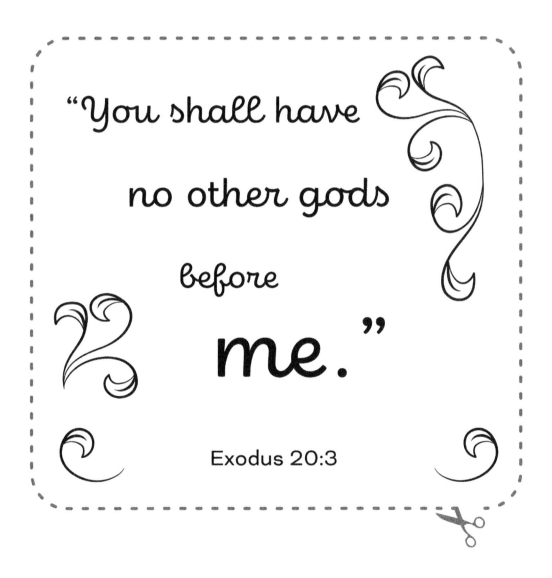

"You shall have no other gods before me."

Exodus 20:3

Journal Your Thoughts

Here is more space to write.

Date: ....

I am thankful for: ....
....
....

Take a "Victory Lap!"

Celebrate success big or small!

Victory Lap: Pause to celebrate your win. Thank the Lord and tell yourself you did a good thing.
Smile and approve of the progress you are making. Enjoy how good it feels. Well done. You did it!!

Date: ....

Victory: ....

How I feel about myself: ....

Why I did it:

Things that helped me succeed:

How God helped me:

I have new hope that:

I could try this strategy again for another win:

What I have learned from the victory:

I am thankful for:

Chapter 9

I'll Do Anything to Get Healthy...
Just Don't Take Away My Ice Cream

What we'll talk about:

Specific foods we "use" to trigger emotional highs.

Why it matters:

"Using" food is a form of substance abuse. When we abuse substances, they abuse us right back.

Wisdom from the Word:

"I'm allowed to do anything, but not everything is helpful. I'm allowed to do anything, but I won't allow anything to gain control over my life."

1 Corinthians 6:12 GWT

Recommended Song of Preparation:

"Walking free" by Micah Tyler

Share a success story about applying Chapter 8 to your life.

_____

_____

_____

_____

Well done!

Binkie Foods

When my husband and I adopted our beautiful twin daughters, they had special needs. Neither would eat. If anything touched their lips, they would vomit. Before we brought them home from the NICU, they needed g-tubes inserted into their stomachs so that we could pour in nutrition. After several months, with much therapy, one of my daughters would accept a pacifier, and that was nothing short of a miracle. Her sister, however, rejected any oral soothing, except her own tiny, curled finger. She did, however, enjoy stealing her sister's pacifier just for the fun of it. She'd inch up to her twin (who wasn't crawling yet), pull out the pacifier, watch her sister cry, and then put it back to stop the crying. Repeat. My daughter had recognized that her twin's sense of peace was tied to the passie, or binky. With it, she was calm; without it, she dissolved into tear-filled fits. My daughter, who was not crawling, grew frustrated with having her pacifier removed. As a result, she was motivated to quickly learn the developmental milestones of crawling and not needing the binky.

There is a time in our life when pacifiers help soothe, but as we mature, we learn to let the pacifier go so that we can grow. Certain foods can be like my daughter's pacifier. When we have them, we are calm, and when we don't, we throw fits. In my own life, I've named these foods my "binky foods." My list has included frosting, pizza, pasta, rice, flour tortillas, and chips. Your list will be different than mine, but the point is all foods are not on the "binky food" list. Most of the time, we have a few specific foods or ingredients, often processed and containing salt, sugar, and fat, that we use to pacify ourselves. My list is small but treacherous because of my need for them.

Are there foods in your life you may be emotionally and/or physically enslaved to?

When you are ready:

   a.   Talk to God about individual foods or ingredients you are leaning on too heavily.

   b.   Write down the name of these foods, and foods God brings to mind as competing with Him as a source of comfort. For example, artichoke dip, vanilla ice cream, and glazed donuts. Not sure how to isolate your idol foods? Ask yourself these questions:

   1.   What unhealthy foods seem impossible to stop eating once I start?

Make a list of foods that come to mind:

_____   _____   _____

_____   _____   _____

   1.   What unhealthy foods, when I eat them, drive me to a string of unhealthy eating decisions? For example: When I eat a tortilla, I want chocolate. After I eat the chocolate, pretzels

sound nice, so I have those. Next, I could really go for a bagel with butter on it … and so on. In other words, once you eat this food, you've lost your footing and slip down a landslide of eating. What foods start these eating binges?

Make a list of foods that come to mind:

_____   _____   _____
_____   _____   _____

2. If this unhealthy food was taken away from me, I'd get mad or deeply sad. I could manage without this food for a day or three, but after a week, I need it, and I don't care who I must push out of the way with my grocery cart to get it. Be specific. Instead of saying "carbs," list specific foods like blueberry muffins. Why? Because it's very possible not all carbs are a problem food, but instead, only a few. An example from my life is that I discovered I don't have a problem with rice in general, but specifically "white sushi rice."

Make a list of foods that come to mind:

_____   _____   _____
_____   _____   _____

3. What are the foods I eat and then hide from God or feel defiant about when it comes to listening to God's guidance concerning how to eat them? In other words, I don't want to talk to God about this food *at all. (God, don't even think about it, I'M NOT giving this food up.)* Yeah, you know the one. Write it below. You can ask God not to look at this part of the page.

Make a list of foods that come to mind:

_____   _____   _____

Nice job considering your trigger foods. If you're like me, it is a sensitive and personal list that might scare you to look at for too long because of how much these foods mean to you. It's okay. Take a deep breath. You can face this, and the Lord is with you to help.

Foods that Block God's Work in Your Life

Pray about removing the unhealthy food(s) on the list from your home and possibly diet for a set time period. Maybe it's mornings; maybe it's just for a day, or one a week.

GASP! How could I suggest such a thing? I know, right. Consider the following:

a. Removing the food will leave an empty space. That void is a place you can practice filling with prayer and subsequently, a relationship with the Lord. As you remember that you want this food desperately-but don't eat it-you are reminded to pray. The longing for the food reminds you to step into the presence of God for help. It's like fasting, but you're still eating healthy food in a healthy way. You're not starving yourself; you're simply removing unhealthy excess foods that have been standing in the way of you going to God first to help you survive daily life.

b.   The food is unhealthy and probably not that great for your body. Removing it for a time may show you that you really don't need it. What if you actually feel better without it? You'll never know if you remove it and realize that you didn't die. (Even though, at times, it might feel on the brink of total devastation.)

Suggestion: Try not eating the unhealthy foods that are stealing your relationship with God for one full day. When you remove the food, replace eating it with prayer when you miss it. If you are truly hungry, have healthy food prepared to eat in its place at the time you normally would eat your unhealthy food. This requires a small amount of food prep that can go a long way toward your health goals.

Oh, Pasta, I Love Thee, Let Me Count the Ways

My personal story (when it comes to making this list) is one of victory, and I'm hoping if you give it a whirl, you get some much needed and satisfying victory in Christ as well.

I'll share with you two foods that were on my list and how I came to work through letting go of them.

The first food on my original list that terrified me to stop eating was white, starchy pasta. I could eat more than a box in a sitting. I refused to discuss it with the Lord for weeks once I realized it was an issue for me. When I did talk to God about it, I cried and cried. With much anger, I followed God's lead and dropped pasta from my diet until I reached my weight goal. Every time I wanted to eat it, I prayed instead and replaced it with a healthy food choice (I now use cauliflower instead of pasta). As time passed, I felt better, lost weight, and now years later, I don't like the taste of pasta, and I don't eat it. It's hard to believe, but I don't want it anymore. I tell you this to let you know that these tricky foods can be overcome. We are not enslaved by anything, not even a food like pasta.

And, you remember how much power frosting had over me.

Can you think of a food that might have too much power over you? While it may be hard to say goodbye to dangerous food, we can do it.

4.   What foods would you grieve to let go of?

_____   _____   _____

5.   Any others you'd like to add?

_____   _____   _____
_____   _____   _____
_____   _____   _____

Breaking Up with Unhealthy Food

When I was struggling with letting go of frosting, I wrote a "break up letter" with frosting. You read my letter in **My Food Story** at the beginning of this book.

Frosting was not healthy for me and looking back, I am so thankful I broke up with this unhealthy, controlling food. Inviting God to help me overcome my love and need for frosting opened up a deeper relationship with Him, which has increased my self-worth and blessed me with better physical and mental health.

Now It's Your Turn

If you have a special food that you are attached to, like I was to frosting, it's understandable. Life is hard, and there are foods that have stood by us when no one else did. Food we thought we could rely on. Food that we need to come to grips with as being harmful and even toxic to our health.

If you have an equivalent of frosting in your life, I want to encourage you to take some time to write a break-up letter with the food. Decide how to separate yourself from the unhealthy relationship with this food for a time so you can regain the sanity and health it may be tampering with. I encourage you to work with Jesus through prayer and listening to His leadership concerning this food regarding when and how you'll consume or not consume it.

When you're ready, write your letter freeform or use the worksheet provided.

Food Break-up Letter

Is there a food that is hurting your heart and your health?
When you're ready, use this worksheet to help you say goodbye.

Dear ....
(Name the food)

Thank you for being there for me.
(Tell the food thanks for being a friend and what it has done for you.)

....

....

....

But now I see that you are harmful to my health
(Tell the food how it is hurting you.)

....

....

....

This is what I need to do
(Talk about how you won't need it or use it anymore and the healthy choices you will make instead.)

....

....

....

I love you, but it's time to break up
(Tell the food goodbye. Share any additional feeings you may have.)

....

....

....

Signed: *Date:*

....

6. Read your letter to the Lord. Give the food and your decision to Him. Write down what comes to mind.

_____
_____
_____
_____
_____
_____
_____
_____
_____
_____
_____
_____
_____

7. Talk to God about your fears, your dreams, and your hopes for a healthier heart, mind, body, and spirit.

_____
_____
_____
_____
_____
_____
_____
_____
_____
_____
_____
_____
_____
_____

8. Ask God to give you a healthy replacement for this food in your life, starting with Him.

_____
_____
_____
_____
_____
_____
_____
_____
_____
_____
_____
_____
_____

Well done. You're on the way to a healthier, happier life journey! YOU DID IT!

Isaiah 43:19:

"See I am doing a new thing! Now it springs up, do you not perceive it? I am making a way in the wilderness and streams in the wasteland."

9.   What new thing do you already see the Lord doing in your life?

_____
_____
_____
_____

What a great break-up letter. You are on your way to freedom from your food strongholds! Excellent work.

Chapter 9 Wrap-Up

10. What is one thing you can do to apply what you learned in this chapter starting today?

_____
_____
_____
_____

Promise Prompt:

Cut this verse out and post it in a place you visit often to remind you that God is helping you overcome unhealthy eating.

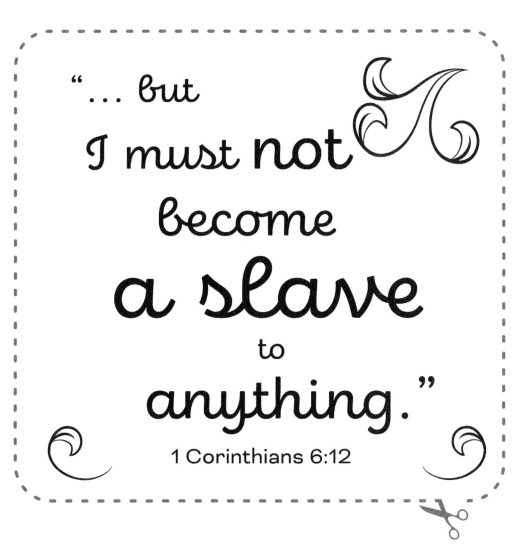

" ... but I must not become a slave to anything."

1 Corinthians 6:12

Journal Your Thoughts

Here is more space to write.

Date: ....

....
....
....
....
....
....
....
....

I am thankful for:..

....

....

Julia Fikse, NBC-HWC, FMCHC

Take a "Victory Lap!"

Celebrate success big or small!

Victory Lap: Pause to celebrate your win. Thank the Lord and tell yourself you did a good thing.
Smile and approve of the progress you are making. Enjoy how good it feels. Well done. You did it!!

Date: ....

Victory: ....

How I feel about myself: ....

Why I did it:
....
....
....

Things that helped me succeed:
....
....

How God helped me:
....
....

I have new hope that:.........................
....

I could try this strategy again for another win:
....

What I have learned from the victory:
....
....

I am thankful for:.........................
....
....

Chapter 10

Please Hold...
The Refrigerator is Calling

What we'll talk about:

Remembering to pray when we are consumed by food.

Why it matters:

Prayer connects us to Jesus, and He can help us stay the course.

Wisdom from the Word:

"But seek ye first His kingdom and His righteousness and all these things shall be added unto you."

Matthew 6:33

Recommended Song of Preparation:

"Battle Belongs" by Phil Wickham

Share a success story about applying Chapter 9 to your life.

_____

_____

_____

_____

Fantastic!

Consuming Food Thoughts

Picture this. I'm standing at the doorway, staring into the dim pantry, eyes locked on the colorful boxes. I inhale the sweet, dusty aroma of cardboard, dry cereal, and wax-coated plastic. You know the smell. I would shut the door and move to this tiny paradise if only it was big enough for a small bed. With my hand thrust in a bent box, I grip a handful of crispy wafers. One tragically breaks in my fist. I can already taste the salt that covers my fingertips.

I am reminded to pray.

OH, MAN! I want these crackers so bad! What am I supposed to do now, put them back? I already touched them; they are mine. Yet, I've been here before (five minutes ago ... same hand, in the same bent box). I already told myself I wasn't going to eat these crackers ... again ... tonight. I'm not hungry, but even if I was, my body would feel better if I ate a healthy snack. I don't want to cut up a carrot. Well, technically, I don't have to cut up a carrot to eat it. But I would have to wash it, maybe. Nah. That would be too much work.

Nevertheless, I had a goal not to eat after 8 p.m. It's what I wanted to do for my health. I've already failed with a handful (or five) of crackers and honestly am not sure if I want to stick to my original plan void of these salty snacks that make my tongue dance.

Who will know anyway?

What's a girl with her hand caught in the cracker box to do?

Eating Is a Spiritual Battle

Read the following verses and think of them in terms of your struggle with food. Consider how eating can be a spiritual battle.

John 10:10

> "The thief's purpose is to steal, kill, and destroy. My purpose is to give life in all its fullness." (Using the word "thief," Jesus is referring to our enemy, Satan.)

1 Peter 5:8

> "Be of sober spirit, be on the alert. Your adversary, the devil, prowls around like a roaring lion, seeking someone to devour."

Ephesians 6:16

> "In addition to all this, take up the shield of faith, with which you can extinguish all the flaming arrows of the evil one."

Psalm 25:15

> "My eyes are ever on the Lord, for only He will release my feet from the snare."

1. With these verses in mind, what does it look like day-to-day, moment-by-moment, to have a *faith in the Lord* that extinguishes spiritual *flaming arrows*? Write some thoughts that come to mind.

_____
_____
_____
_____
_____
_____
_____
_____
_____
_____
_____
_____

When the crumbs are flying in a spiritual battle for our health, everyday consistent, small decisions matter (as well as the big ones). Therefore, we need a plan of action to get with God quickly and ask for His power to help. Here's a tool, in the form of an acronym, you can use to get out of tricky food situations and back on your plan for your health with God's help.

Let's "STAY LOW"

STAY LOW is an acronym we can use to remind us how to practically get with God and get out of the way of harmful food and damaging food behaviors.

STAY LOW
 Seek Him
 Trust Him
 Ask Him
 Yes, Lord
 Listen
 Obey Him
 Watch Him work

STAY LOW is ***not*** a fear-based hiding mentality. Instead, the goal is to seek God and shelter with Him, trusting that He will come to the rescue and give you the strength and wisdom you need to stand strong with Him by your side.

We *are not* afraid.
We *are* regrouping and taking refuge in the Lord, His presence, His wisdom, and His strength.

"The LORD himself will fight for you. Just stay calm."
Exodus 14:14

S: Seek Him

Our first step to successfully finding our help in Christ when it comes to our food challenges is to seek Him *first*. What does this look like practically?

We begin by making a deliberate decision to stop seeking out food and change course to seek God. Walk away from the food and go to the Lord instead. Go with empty hands and an empty mouth. Cease the action of unhealthy eating (or intent to eat unhealthily) and talk to Jesus before filling up with food.

Matthew 6:33

> "But seek ye first the kingdom of God, and his righteousness; and all these things shall be added unto you."

Worried you won't remember to go to God in the moment? Ask the Holy Spirit to help you! I ask the Holy Spirit when I remember to remind me when I don't remember. Our flesh is weak, and our memory is short, but the Holy Spirit gives us the strength and recall we need to act wisely for the sake of our physical and mental well-being.

John 14:26

> "But the Helper, the Holy Spirit, whom the Father will send in My name, He will teach you all things, and bring to your remembrance all things that I said to you."

Prayer allows the Holy Spirit into your mind to help manage your thoughts, decisions, and desires before breaking into the old habits of unhealthy eating. Seeking Him is the first step.

2. Write about how "seeking Jesus" before seeking unhealthy food might help you reach your healthy eating goals.

_____
_____
_____
_____
_____
_____
_____
_____
_____
_____
_____
_____
_____
_____
_____
_____

T: Trust Him

Believe that God is good, and He *will* help you.

Hebrews 11:6 says:

> "And without faith it is impossible to please God, because anyone who comes to Him must believe that He exists and that He rewards those who earnestly seek Him."

Once we put food aside, let's pause and trust the Lord with what we are facing. We can trust Him with our food, our heart, and a circumstance that may be causing our "food drivers" to ignite a desire to eat instead of praying. God can help us overcome powerful emotions so that we can approach food with perspective and reason.

Romans 8:28 says:

> "And we know that all things work together for good to them that love God and are called according to His purpose."

3. Tell a story about a time God was trustworthy in your life.

4. Write about how remembering this experience helps you trust the Lord when it comes to deciding what to eat and how to eat.

A: Ask Him for help.

What does "asking God for help" practically look like in the moment? *Immediate short prayer.* My emergency prayers are shot like arrows straight to my source of power and often go something like this:

"Jesus, help."
"God, I need you."
"Lord, please!"

As you can see, no brilliant, amazing, earth-shattering prayers here. I've learned they don't need to be fancy. Simply call on the Lord. As we studied earlier, He wants to help you, He will help you, and He knows how to help you fast.

5.   What short prayer could you pray when you are surrounded by food and need help?

_____
_____
_____
_____
_____
_____

Y: Yes, Lord.

We are in the best place to receive a word from the Holy Spirit when we have already agreed to listen to His voice. Saying "Yes, Lord, I'm listening" is about being open to the idea of adjusting from what we want to what God shares is best.

Jesus gave us the ultimate example. He asked God to take death on the cross away if possible. He prayed this simple, humble, faith-filled prayer of willingness and submission.

Mark 14:36

"Not my will, but yours be done."

Willingness is a difficult step. However, with practice, this muscle of faith grows, and in time, it does become stronger. It gets easier. When we feel discouraged, we may go back to our old habits. But let's not grow weary of doing good; there is no better person to say "yes" to than our loving, living Lord.

6.   To what request is the Lord asking you to say "yes" when it comes to your health?

_____
_____
_____
_____
_____
_____
_____

7. How might saying "Yes, Lord" help you realize your healthy eating goals?

_____
_____
_____
_____
_____
_____
_____
_____
_____

L: Listen

Now it's time to listen to how the Holy Spirit may guide you. A word from the Lord will always be in line with the Word of God found in the Bible. It may be a still, small voice you hear from your heart, an encouragement that comes from another person, a scripture verse or song, or something that comes another way. The Lord is very creative and knows how to get our attention.

Psalm 34:4

> "I sought the LORD and He answered me, and rescued me from all my fears."

1 Corinthians 10:13 says:

> "No temptation has overtaken you except what is common to mankind. And God is faithful; He will not let you be tempted beyond what you can bear. But when you are tempted, He will also provide a way out so that you can endure it."

Put this verse into practice by asking God for a way out and listening for an answer from the Holy Spirit.

8. Share a story about how you asked the Lord for help, and He provided a way out of an eating challenge.

For example, "I was at a party with a buffet, and I was terrified I would lose control, but the Lord allowed a friend to come over and talk with me. We had a great conversation, and I was completely distracted from the food table."

_____
_____
_____
_____
_____
_____
_____
_____
_____

O: Obey

The Lord is wonderfully creative and may bring to light a helpful idea or Bible verse as you pray. Following the guidance of the Holy Spirit, which will always be grounded in Scripture, is a practical way to stay on your healthy course to take care of your body.

God's help is a gift. It may feel like discipline or be uncomfortable to follow His guidance. Obeying God can feel very risky. Experiencing His goodness through the door of obedience makes it easier to follow Him the next time. Obedience is tough because it often means not doing what we want. But … what if what we want to do isn't going to serve us? God knows what is best for us and He won't lead us astray.

Proverbs 14:12 says:

"There is a way that appears to be right, but in the end, it leads to death."

Ephesians 4:27 says:

"… and give no opportunity to the devil."[2]

When we eat food that we know is not good for our bodies, that food is harmful to our physical well-being and can lead us to death.

Ask yourself, "Are my eating habits leading me to greater life?" Let's explore.

9. What eating do you practice that leads to life?

_____
_____
_____
_____
_____
_____
_____

10. What eating do you practice that leads to death? Add details about how the food or practice leads to physical, spiritual, or emotional death.

_____
_____
_____
_____
_____
_____
_____

---

[2] The context for this verse is anger, but there are some food-related eating patterns that can give the devil an opportunity to harm us.

God wants us to have an abundant life, which can be affected negatively or positively by our food choices.

11. What does God know about you that He might be considering when He offers healthy solutions for you and your life specifically?

_____

_____

_____

_____

_____

_____

12. How might following the Lord's instructions when it comes to food consumption lead to an abundant life?

_____

_____

_____

_____

_____

There can be a cost to following God … but He is faithful. He knows what will bless *your* life and how to help you step into that blessing. Sometimes we must obey *before* being blessed, which can be scary and uncomfortable.

John 1:16

"From His abundance we have all received one gracious blessing after another."

Write down some examples of how you follow God in your life. For example, I donate to my church even though I'd rather keep the money, or I make baskets for foster kids because God wants me to help people in need, or I always tell the truth because God wants us to be honest.

13. Share a story about a time you followed the Lord and were blessed as a result.

_____

_____

_____

_____

_____

14. How does remembering God's blessing encourage you to follow Him when it comes to your eating choices?

_____

_____

_____

_____

_____

_____

_____

W: Watch

Over the next several days, watch how God works in your life. Each time you want to reach for something unhealthy and decide to pray, what comes to mind? What did the Lord put in your head? We must watch for His providence, or it may fly right by us, and we don't want to miss it! Let's be watchful of the Lord as He is working in our lives.

Use this space to record what the Lord does to help you overcome unhealthy eating as you STAY LOW.

Date: _____
What God Did:

_____
_____
_____ Date: _____

What God Did:

_____
_____
_____ Date: _____

What God Did:

_____
_____
_____ Date: _____

15. What is one thing you can do to apply what you learned in this chapter starting today?

_____
_____
_____
_____

Promise Prompt:

Cut this verse out and post it in a place you visit often to remind you that God is helping you overcome unhealthy eating.

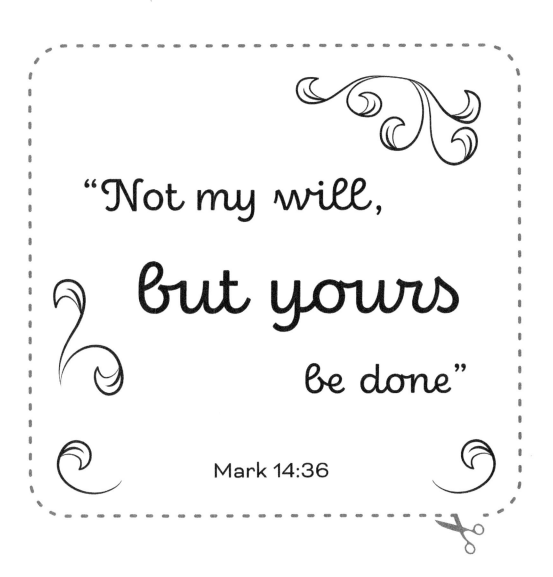

"Not my will, but yours be done"

Mark 14:36

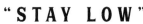

"STAY LOW"

Seek Him
Trust Him
Ask Him
YES, Lord
Listen
Obey Him
Watch Him work

"STAY LOW"

Seek Him
Trust Him
Ask Him
YES, Lord
Listen
Obey Him
Watch Him work

"STAY LOW"

SEEK HIM
TRUST HIM
ASK HIM
YES, LORD
LISTEN
OBEY HIM
WATCH HIM WORK

"STAY LOW"

Seek Him
Trust Him
Ask Him
YES, Lord
Listen
Obey Him
Watch Him work

"STAY LOW"

Seek Him
Trust Him
Ask Him
YES, Lord
Listen
Obey Him
Watch Him work

"STAY LOW"

SEEK HIM
TRUST HIM
ASK HIM
YES, LORD
LISTEN
OBEY HIM
WATCH HIM WORK

"STAY LOW"

Seek Him
Trust Him
Ask Him
YES, Lord
Listen
Obey Him
Watch Him work

"STAY LOW"

Seek Him
Trust Him
Ask Him
YES, Lord
Listen
Obey Him
Watch Him work

"STAY LOW"

SEEK HIM
TRUST HIM
ASK HIM
YES, LORD
LISTEN
OBEY HIM
WATCH HIM WORK

Journal Your Thoughts

Here is more space to write.

Date: ....

....
....
....
....
....
....
....
....

I am thankful for: ....
....
....

Take a "Victory Lap!"

Celebrate success big or small!

Victory Lap: Pause to celebrate your win. Thank the Lord and tell yourself you did a good thing.
Smile and approve of the progress you are making. Enjoy how good it feels. Well done. You did it!!

Date: ....

Victory: ....

How I feel about myself: ....

Why I did it:
....
....
....
....

Things that helped me succeed:
....
....
....

How God helped me:
....
....

I have new hope that:................
....

I could try this strategy again for another win:
....

What I have learned from the victory:
....
....

I am thankful for:................
....
....

Congratulations!

You've completed Workbook One.

Way to go!

Now that food is off the throne, we'll need systems and strategies to keep it off.

Welcome to Workbook Two.

I can't wait.

See you there.

Acknowledgements

First, much love and gratitude to my husband Craig, and my daughters for their love, patience, and support. Also, thank you Craig for stepping in and helping when I was at my wits end… for example: going out and ordering a cake with me, taking the cover photo, and making the frosting strawberry flavor (ew gross!) so I wouldn't want to eat it. You're amazing, Craig Fikse.

Many thanks and appreciation to: Sky Rodio Nuttall my talented editor, Kim Houser for the final proof-read, and Casey Sharpe, who helped make my worksheets pretty. Also, to my friend and nutritionist, Heather Wood, for holding me accountable to logging my food, banishing shame, and eat intentionally for health and well-being.

And to my early readers: treasured friends and family who took time out of their busy lives to read a chapter, or a draft, share their honest feedback, and encourage me to keep going. My sincere thanks to each one for their valuable contribution to this project.

Kara Adame
Jennifer Baham
Cheryl Bean
Gina Biri
Kim Bracken
Mary Caballero
Kathy Carder
Julia Carter
Roslyn Casterline
Susan Chavez
Jamie DiLuigi
Lindsay Downs
Lyndy Downs
Michelle Emard
David Field
Nicole Field
Craig Fikse
Barbara Funk
Michelle Gerard

Alicia Gibson
Christine Hawkins
Sharon Hagen
Lynn Johnson
Karmen Karatsonyi
Chris Lansdown
Tricia Lawley
Mary Matsuno
Maria Mohrman
Monica Origer
Pamela Rumph
Lara Scheel
Terry Skarpelli
Christina Stalboeger
Julie Thurber
Dori Yenokian
Michael Yearley
Heather Yonkers

Julia Fikse loves speaking!

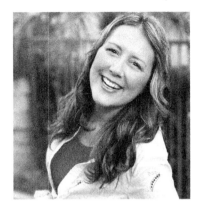

To request Julia to speak at your group or event
in person or online, please reach out through the contact
form at:
www.onesteptowellness.com

Julia has over 25 years of speaking experience and would
love to personally encourage your community through:

-live events
-online events
-podcasts
-radio interviews
-workshops
-retreats
-and more!

Book Julia today!

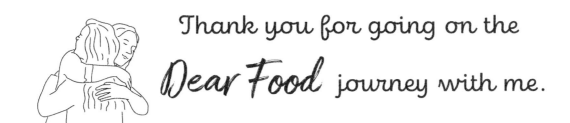

Thank you for going on the *Dear Food* journey with me.

If this book has helped you
overcome food strongholds, please bless others by
leaving a review on Amazon.

The more positive reviews this book receives,
the more Amazon will share it with those seeking support
to overcome their food challenges.
Thank you!

If you have feedback you believe would be helpful to
improve the material, please contact me
personally so that I can address your comments and
concerns directly.

I value your input to make this book and my future books better.

You can reach me through the contact form at:
www.onesteptowellness.com

Thank you! - Julia Fikse

Printed in Great Britain
by Amazon

42066783R00119